IPP Studies in the Frontiers of China's Public Policy

Series Editor

Feng Zhang, South China University of Technology, Guangzhou, China

IPP Studies in the Frontiers of China's Public Policy combines original research and theoretical innovation to provide fresh insights into the fast-changing landscape of China's public policy. Books in the series, written by scholars based inside China or commissioned by the IPP, draw on local Chinese experiences to generate empirical findings and theoretical insights. The field of China's public policy is broadly defined to include all aspects of the country's social, economic, technological and foreign policies. The series encourage interdisciplinary approaches to public policy, with a special but not exclusive focus on the study of south China, especially the Guangdong, Hong Kong, Macau Greater Bay Area, one of the most vibrant regions of growth and innovation in China.

Liu Jia

Obligation

The Changing Physician-Patient Relationship and Healthcare Reforms in China

palgrave
macmillan

Liu Jia
South China University
of Technology
Guangzhou, China

IPP Studies in the Frontiers of China's Public Policy
ISBN 978-981-99-6436-9 ISBN 978-981-99-6437-6 (eBook)
https://doi.org/10.1007/978-981-99-6437-6

Cover credit: Jake Olimb/Gettyimages

This Palgrave Macmillan imprint is published by the registered company Springer Nature Singapore Pte Ltd.
The registered company address is: 152 Beach Road, #21-01/04 Gateway East, Singapore 189721, Singapore

Paper in this product is recyclable.

Acknowledgments

The physician–patient relationship has been widely discussed in academic research. Most legal and ethical studies approach it from the perspective of rights. However, as this book has tried to show, it is obligations rather than rights that deeply shape our interactions with others. As this book was being written, the world was ravaged by the Covid-19 pandemic. The outbreak of such an unprecedented pandemic invites us to reconsider our relationship with others: can we find the "common good" in a pandemic? A reflection on this question requires us to probe into how we define what is best for the health of the most people and how to realize the right to health in the least heartless way. These are the particular questions that have perplexed me while writing this book.

In order to be able to complete this book, I would first of all like to express my sincere and heartfelt gratitude to Professor Scott Veitch, Professor Zheng Yongnian, and Professor Zhang Feng. Their knowledge and intelligence nurture my research ability, their attitude toward research influences my understanding of knowledge, and most importantly, their virtues of generosity and humility shape my character as a potential scholar.

I would also like to express my sincere gratitude to other teachers and friends, Dr. Li Jie, Professor Li Haibin, Professor Jiang Yuhao, Dr. Guo Hai, Dr. Yang Haiyan, Dr. Zhang Jun, and Dr. Wang Qi who have encouraged and supported me at various stages. Without their encouragement, I might not be so determined to continue my research in medical ethics and law. I am also very grateful for the efforts of Dr. Jacob Dreyer of Palgrave Macmillan. I also deeply appreciate the hard work and kind help of our faculty staff, especially Ms. Wang Yan, Ms. Zhouying, and Ms. Liang Hailing.

An earlier version of Chapter 3 has been published in *Asian Journal of Law and Society*. An earlier version of Chapter 6 has been published in *Human Security in China: A Post-Pandemic State* edited by Dr. Chi Zhang.

Contents

List of Charts

List of Tables

CHAPTER 1

Introduction

Beijing physician Tao Yong, a 40-year-old physician, the head of ophthalmology at Beijing, was brutally pierced by a patient in the head and arm in January 2020. In another case, Hu Shuyun, a cardiologist in Jiangxi Province, was stabbed by a male suspect surnamed Zeng in January 2021. The National Health Commission issued a statement afterward, calling for the attention of all society to protect the life and safety of medical professionals, maintain medical order, as well as protect the rights of physicians and patients. Physician–patient relationship, which denotes "*yihuan guanxi*" (醫患關係) in Chinese, has been widely discussed in academic research, mass media, and everyday discussions. This relationship not only refers to the one between physicians and patients to improve the health and welfare of patients, but also involves relatives of patients as well as other medical professionals, such as health officials and nurses. The physician–patient relationship is rife with conflicting interests and personal experiences, various social-economic forces, and different institutional norms.

Most studies address the decline of trust in the physician–patient relationship by investigating patients' and physicians' *rights*, expectations, and experiences. Rights, especially the specification and pursuit of patients' rights, have been widely discussed in the legislation and literature of healthcare and medical laws in China. The basic medical and healthcare law, i.e., Law of People's Republic of China on the Promotion of

L. Jia, *Obligation*, IPP Studies in the Frontiers of China's Public Policy,
https://doi.org/10.1007/978-981-99-6437-6_1

Basic Medical and Healthcare (基本醫療衛生與健康促進法) (hereinafter "Basic Health Law") promulgated on December 28, 2019, specifies both patients' rights—including the right to healthcare, the right to informed consent, the right to privacy, etc.—and physicians' rights—including the right to life, the right to security, the right to dignity, other physicians' rights recognized under the rule of law, etc. The discussions enumerating and pursuing rights cover access to healthcare, privacy, truth-telling, and informed consent together with criminal and civil litigations and remedies.[1] The recognition of patients' rights in China not only involves the practice or implementation of the legal norms, but concerns the conflicts and interactions between the legal norms and Chinese cultural traditions.[2] The discussions on the advancement of patients' rights also call for attention to their correlatives of duties.[3] For instance, the right to informed consent generates the duties of improving the communication skills of medical professionals, reforming the current market-based healthcare system, and formulating and implementing related social policies essential to fully protect patients' rights.[4]

[1] *See* Ruiping Fan & Benfu Li, "Truth Telling in Medicine: The Confucian View," *The Journal of Medicine and Philosophy: A Forum for Bioethics and Philosophy of Medicine* 29(2), 2004; Jingchun Cao, "Protecting the Right to Privacy in China," *Victoria University of Wellington Law Review* 645; Xiju Zhao, "Chinese Medical Negligence Law: How to Distinguish and Accommodate Common Law Principles?," in Lei Chen and Cornelis Hendrik van Rhee, eds., *Toward a Chinese Civil Code*, Leiden: Martius Nijhoff Publishers, 2012; Zhu Wang & Ken Oliphant, "Yangge Dance: The Rhythm of Liability for Medical Malpractice in the People's Republic of China," *Chicago-Kent Law Review* 87(1), 2012; "Claims, Liabilities, Injures and Compensation Payments of Medical Malpractice Litigation Cases in China from 1998 to 2011," *BMC Health Services Research* 14, 2014; Benjamin Liebman, "Malpractice Mobs: Medical Dispute Resolution in China," *Columbia Law Review* 113, 2013.

[2] *See* Jing-Bao Nie, *Medical Ethics in China: A Transcultural Interpretation*, London: Routledge, 2013; Yongfu Cao, Yunling Wang & Linjuan Zheng, "Towards a Confucian Approach to Health Care Allocation in China: A Dynamic Geography," in *China: Bioethics, Trust, and the Challenge of the Market*, 2008; Raposo Vera Lúcia, "Lost in 'Culturation': Medical Informed Consent in China (From a Western Perspective)," *Medicine, Health Care and Philosophy* 22, 2019.

[3] Yang Lixin & Yuan Xueshi, "On the Medical Organization's Tort Liability of Violating the Obligation of Informed Consent," *Hebei Law Science* 2006.

[4] Jing-Bao Nie, "Is Informed Consent Not Applicable to China? Intellectual Flaws of the 'Cultural Difference Argument'," *Formosan Journal of Medical Humanities* 2(2), 2001.

Despite the large number of patients' and physicians' rights, in recent years China has witnessed a surge in medical disputes and intense conflicts between physicians and patients. The total number of medical disputes has been rising by 22.9% each year since 2002. Each hospital deals with 27 cases of medical violence targeted at physicians every year. The total number of violent cases targeting medical professionals jumped from 10,248 in 2006 to 17,243 in 2010.[5] Once respected as "angels in white", medical professionals are facing unprecedented challenges. A survey revealed that only 26% of physicians found their patients trusted them.[6] In this sense, although there have been a growing number of patients' and physicians' rights, both physicians and patients feel they are vulnerable to the other side and there has been a decline in physician–patient trust. Most studies address the decline of trust in the physician–patient relationship by investigating patients' and physicians' rights, as well as their expectations, experiences, and the societal, institutional, and interpersonal factors eroding their trust.

The discussions enumerating and pursuing rights cover access to healthcare, privacy, truth-telling, and informed consent together with criminal and civil litigations and remedies. The recognition of patients' rights in China not only involves the practice or implementation of the legal norms, but concerns the conflicts and interactions between the legal norms and Chinese cultural traditions. The key issue under the discussions is whether Western values, such as individual autonomy promoted by the doctrine of informed consent, are alien and incompatible with the Chinese cultural and moral traditions which are commonly described as communitarian, emphasizing the significance of the state, community, and family instead of the individual. The discussions on the advancement of patients' rights also call for attention to their correlative duties. For instance, the right to informed consent generates physician obligations to inform patients of illness condition, items for examination, principles of treatment, potential danger of different treatments, recommendations

[5] Alex Jingwei He & Jiwei Qian, "Explaining Medical Disputes in Chinese Public Hospitals: The Doctor-Patient Relationship and its Implications for Health Policy Reforms," *Health, Economy, Policy and Law* 11, 2016, pp. 362–3.

[6] Ibid., 362.

on the treatment plans, items to be concerned about during and after hospitalization, the time for follow-up examinations, and the like.[7]

The writing on healthcare in China also revolves around the deteriorated trust in physicians. A societal moral decline in the post-Mao era, together with the healthcare system's orientation toward profit-making, the financing mechanism of public hospitals, the income structure of physicians, as well as the attitudes and manners in which physicians and patients communicate with each other, have been identified as the societal, institutional, and interpersonal factors eroding the trust between physicians and patients.[8] Law and legal institutions have also been recognized as not providing incentives for hospitals to reduce medical malpractice.[9] Ethical and legal suggestions to rebuild physician–patient trust thus require reforming not only China's flawed healthcare system, but the social and legal institutions more fundamentally.[10]

Culture and bioethics studies have emphasized their primacy of morality and ethics in medicine practices. Studies of cultural factors tend to provide important information and details on the operation of social practices and customs of medicine in China. While the sociological and anthropologist studies of medicine in contemporary China do

[7] Yali Cong, "Doctor–Family–Patient Relationship: The Chinese Paradigm of Informed Consent," *Journal of Medicine and Philosophy: A Forum for Bioethics and Philosophy* 29, 2004, p. 154.

[8] *See* Cheris Shun-ching Chan, "Mistrust of Physicians in China: Society, Institutions, and Interaction as Root Causes," *Developing World Bioethics* 18, 2018, pp. 16–25; Benjamin L. Liebman, "Law in the Shadow of Violence: Can Law Help to Improve Doctor–Patient Trust in China?," *Columbia Journal of Asian Law* 30, 2016, pp. 113–30; Jing-Bao Nie, Lun Li, Grant Gillett, Joseph D. Tucker & Arthur Kleinman, "The Crisis of Patient–Physician Trust and Bioethics: Lessons and Inspirations from China," *Developing World Bioethics* 18, 2018, pp. 56–64; Jing-Bao Nie, Yu Cheng, Xiang Zou, et al., "The Vicious Circle of Patient–Physician Mistrust in China: Health Professionals' Perspectives, Institutional Conflict of Interest, and Building Trust Through Medical Professionalism," *Developing World Bioethics* 18, 2018, pp. 26–36; Xiang Zou, Yu Cheng & Jing-Bao Nie, "The Social Practice of Medical Guanxi (Personal Connections) and Patient–Physician Trust in China: An Anthropological and Ethical Study," *Developing World Bioethics* 18, 2018, pp. 45–55.

[9] Benjamin L. Liebman, "Law in the Shadow of Violence: Can Law Help to Improve Doctor–Patient Trust in China?," *Columbia Journal of Asian Law* 30, 2016, pp. 113–30.

[10] Joseph D. Tucker, Bonnie Wong, Jing-Bao Nie & Arthur Kleinman, "Rebuilding Patient–Physician Trust in China," *The Lancet* 388, 2016, p. 755.

not seek to offer a critical or normative analysis, they produce an ethnography that demonstrates ethical pluralism as an intrinsic aspect of Chinese medical practice.[11] German medical anthropologist Volker Scheid points out that Chinese medicine "is not a totality... reducible to a singular cultural logic or process of production".[12] Scheid's analysis of Chinese Medicine in contemporary China explains the formation of the Chinese medicine by multiple factors, or "infrastructures", including physicians, patients, disease syndromes, and the state. The analysis offers a cultural background, which helps bioethics studies to make informed ethical judgments on their practices. As noted by Nie Jingbao, "[e]ngaged interpretations are essential to any normative judgment. *Either* simply applying normative ethical principles developed within a particular moral tradition to cross-cultural settings *or* merely respecting cultural differences and the particularity of the local is both practically dangerous and theoretically problematic".[13]

This book adopts the approach developed by Allan Hutchinson which seeks to "resurface the politics and history presently submerged in the enterprise" of medical law. This approach differs from the dominant discussions among medical law scholars, which posit bioethics as a higher standard against which legislative and judicial developments must be tested. According to the dominant views, medical law and legal developments must be examined to determine whether they are consistent with or reflect standards set by medical ethics or bioethics.[14] For instance, as will be explained in this book, the right to informed consent is called on to ensure that patient autonomy is given appropriate respect and protection as understood in different ethical theories. The doctrine of informed consent, as well as specific decisions regarding administrative and civil liabilities is evaluated in accordance with the ethical principles of patient autonomy. The concrete principles of medical ethics vary, as they may come from different traditions, such as Western liberalism and Eastern Confucianism. Notwithstanding these differences, they share congruence

[11] *See* for instance Volker Scheid, *Chinese Medicine in Contemporary China: Plurality and Synthesis*, Durham, NC: Duke University Press, 2002.

[12] Ibid., 13.

[13] Jing-Bao Nie, *Medical Ethics in China: A Transcultural Interpretation*, London: Routledge, 2011, p. 12.

[14] *See* John Harrington, *Towards a Rhetoric of Medical Law: Against Ethics*, Abingdon, Oxon: Routledge, 2016, chapter 1.

in certain basic principles of ethics and their subordination to the principles of ethics. Different from the dominant views, this book takes the approach to exploring how the doctrines of medical ethics and law interact as rhetoric with each other.

Rhetoric is, as noted by Peter Goodrich,

> political criticism in its classical sense of the study of arguments related to the historical situation and immediate needs of the community (*polis*) to which the speech or discourse is addressed.[15]

This view presents us a number of implications. It directs us to explore how the "historical situation" has affected the relations between citizens in "the community", as well as the "needs" of the community. This is not an objective reflection of the characteristics of the community and their needs. Instead, it is a constitutive process of understanding and determining the purposes and needs of the community as well as defining their history. Deploying the analysis taken by Harrington, this book discusses the ethical and legal speech as a "locus of historical conflict", which works as a site of a power struggle between different notions of the community, its needs, and the relationship with the law.[16] Thus, this book investigates the historical processes by which different values and the community have been constituted. It considers the assumptions and strategies by which certain groups achieve authority and credibility.

In addition, there is a large body of literature on patients' rights that leaves two related questions unresolved. First, can the discourse of rights provide the best perspective for observing the social relations—in particular, trust, mistrust, or distrust—between physicians and patients, between citizens and the state? Secondly, can the relations between physicians and patients be observed independently of other forms of relations, i.e., relations between citizens and the state? The answers to these two questions, as explained in this book, will lead to a better observation and explanation of how social practices and social institutions function in the field of health care.

[15] Peter Goodrich, *Reading the Law: A Critical Introduction to Legal Method and Critiques*, New York, NY: Blackwell, 1986, pp. 171–2.

[16] Roland Barthes, *The Semiotic Challenge*, Berkeley, CA: University of California Press, 1994, p. 47.

This book takes a perspective that examines obligations rather than rights in health care. Specifically, it examines the issue of physician–patient obligation in the context of China's healthcare reform. By considering the physician–patient relationship as an essential part of the public health system, this book explores the relationship between obligation and the changing nature of the public health system in China. China's healthcare reform has been ongoing for decades. Since the founding of the PRC in 1949, it has gone through three stages: a combination of government-funded health care in urban areas and community health care in rural areas before 1978, a market-oriented healthcare reform between 1978 and 2002, and the current round of healthcare reform after 2002. Against this background, this book presents an observation and analysis of the changing nature and function of physician–patient obligations.

To provide a better perspective of the foregoing observation, this book draws on recent jurisprudential work, which challenges the once-settled understanding of the equal relations between rights and obligations. Jeremy Waldron argues that when rights are considered, even negative rights, they generate multiple kinds of obligations rather than a single form of obligations.[17] Onora O'Neill also notes this point in the context of social and economic rights, arguing that the focus on rights obscures the essential work done by claims about obligations which make rights effective, such as specifying "not only what is to be accorded, but which obligation-bearers are going to have to do what for whom and at what cost".[18] This is because it is obligations rather than rights that are closely related to the work done by the contributor, the producer, and the active citizen. As put by O'Neill: "It takes the perspective of the claimant rather than of the contributor, of the consumer rather than of the producer, of the passive rather than the active citizen".[19] Thus, Scott Veitch further observes that "[e]mphasising the second of each of these pairs—contributor, producer, active citizen—requires a sustained commitment to harness multiple (waves of) duties and responsibilities in a complex set of engagements that is too-easily underplayed in the

[17] Jeremy Waldron, "Rights in Conflict," *Ethics* 99(3), 1989, pp. 503–19.

[18] Onora O'Neill, "Women's Rights: Whose Obligations?," in *Bounds of Justice*, Cambridge; New York: Cambridge University Press, 2000, p. 100.

[19] Ibid., 101.

commonplace proclamation of a 'rights culture'".[20] What is emphasized here is that it is obligations, and in particular "waves of duties" rather than rights, that can best capture our understanding of social practices.

In addition to the correlative account of obligations and rights, Scott Veitch also explores how the bond or tie lies at the core of obligation. As put by Scott Veitch, "this sense of tying or binding is a central component of understanding social and professional obligations, and indeed social and professional life".[21] In the particular context of the National Health Service (hereinafter "NHS"), Kenneth Veitch draws on the idea of Alain Supiot and others that the bond lies at the heart of obligation's etymology and offers a historical analysis of the obligations, through which he analyzes not only the substantive obligations but also the shifting nature of obligations and the bond between physicians and patients as well as that between the citizen and the state. Drawing on the above ideas and inspirations, this book is not only interested in examining the changing types of substantive obligation, but also in analyzing the shifting ties and bonds that underpin the physician–patient relationship as well as the citizen–state relationship. It also analyzes the roles played by law and legal institutions—the laws that implement the notion of informed consent, the right to health, and provide for tort liability—in facilitating the changing nature of the obligations.

This book also discusses the concept of trust to understand how the trusting relations may be established between physicians and patients. According to Annette Baier, trust refers to an expectation of benefiting from others' goodwill.[22] The idea of trust is the bedrock on which social relations and other values are built. As Sisela Bok remarks, "[i]f there is no confidence in the truthfulness of others, is there any way to assess their fairness, their intensions to help or to harm? How, then, can they be trusted? Whatever matters to human beings, trust is the atmosphere in which it thrives".[23] Niklaus Luhmann also observes a conceptual link between trust and vulnerability in the sense that trust is viewed as a way of

[20] Scott Veitch, "Sense of Obligation," *Jurisprudence* 8(3), 2017, p. 423.

[21] Ibid., 416.

[22] Annette Baier, "Trust and Antitrust," *Ethics* 96, 1986, pp. 234–5.

[23] Sissela Bok, *Secrets: On the Ethics of Concealment and Revelation*, New York: Pantheon Books, 1982, p. 31.

overcoming the uncertainties that the future contains.[24] The uncertainties and vulnerability about the future explain the necessity of trust for interpersonal relationships and for quality health care. In the medical context, trust is defined by Marsh and Dibben as a belief that the trusted would "act in the best interests of another (the truster) in a given situation, even when controls are unavailable and it may not be in the trustee's best interests to do so".[25] Four dimensions of trust are crucial between physicians and patients, including, fidelity, competency, honesty, and confidentiality of physicians.[26] The trust between them can thus be broken through deliberate fault or incompetence.

This book consists of seven chapters. After the introduction, the second chapter explores the types of factors that have contributed to the formation of barefoot physicians' sense of ethical obligation. This chapter also identifies the connection between the collective nature of healthcare and physicians' ethical sense of obligation. The analysis then turns to explore how the doctrine of informed consent and the right to health, as typical examples of Western medical ethics, have been incorporated and developed in contemporary China. The first part of the third chapter examines some of the literature on the introduction of informed consent into the Chinese healthcare context that seeks to ground the ethical senses of physician and patient obligation as required by the notion of informed consent. The second part analyzes how the right to health has been conceived in China. In the fourth chapter, this book analyzes how health policy and medical law, in the context of the marketization of health care, have contributed to the decoupling of physicians' and patients' practices from their ethical sense of obligation. Then, in the fifth chapter, the book examines the effects of the current round of healthcare reform on physicians' and patients' practices of obligation. Through an analysis of a number of examples—including public hospital reform, public contracting, and tort liability in the area of informed consent—the aim is

[24] Niklas Lumann, *Trust and Power: Two Works by Niklas Luhmann*, Chichester, New York, Brisbane, Toronto: John Wiley & Sons, 1982, pp. 12–23.

[25] Stephen Marsh & Mark Dibben, "Trust, Untrust, Distrust and Mistrust—An Exploration of the Dark(er) Side," in P. Hermann, V. Issarny & S. Shui, eds., *Trust Management*, Berlin: Springer, 2005, p. 19.

[26] Yunxiang Yan, "The Ethics and Politics of Patient-Physician Mistrust in Contemporary China," *Developing World Bioethics* 18, 2018, p. 8.

to mark a shift away from the barefoot doctors' sense of ethical obligation and a decoupling from the physician's and patient's sense of ethical obligation as set forth in the healthcare reform plan. The sixth chapter traces the emergence and development of the legal and regulatory scheme of public health emergency management in China. Using the Covid-19 pandemic, the SARS crisis, and the patriotic hygiene campaigns in the 1950s as three examples, this chapter analyzes how law and legal institutions have functioned in response to major public health emergencies in China and reveals a potential decline in people's trust in public hospitals. This book finally turns to the discussions regarding how to bring trust back to the physician–patient relationship in China and proposes that the legal doctrine of informed consent should be reconfigured through fiduciary law to strengthen the physician obligations of care taking as well as patient obligations of experience and story sharing.

CHAPTER 2

Historical Background: Barefoot Doctor Program

After the foundation of People's Republic of China in 1949, similar to its Nationalist predecessor, the Communist government was committed to modernization.[1] At a general level, since World War II, policymakers around the world had hubristically believed that the international system could be operated and manipulated to achieve their own objectives. Since the late 1960s, this was no longer the case. The 1970s witnessed the decline of the consensus on the dominant Western values since World War II. Across the Western world, the 1970s provided ideological inclination to conservatives. Margaret Thatcher, Ronald Reagan, and Jeane Kirkpatrick were those individuals who had accepted the liberal norms but began to embrace free market theory and deregulation at home and extend the anti-communist line in international affairs.[2] The Western officials assertively sought to supervise the rest of the world to accept political and economic transitions. The 1970s also witnessed a period of optimism about what the international order should be achieved in decolonized nations. These nations were considering how political independence could

[1] *See* Ka-che Yip, *Health and National Reconstruction in Nationalist China, The Development of Modern Health Services, 1928–1937*, Ann Arbor, Michigan: Association for Asian Studies, 1995, p. 6.

[2] Richard Vinen, *Thatcher's Britain: The Politics and Social Upheaval of the 1980s*, London: Simon & Schuster, Limited 2010.

L. Jia, *Obligation*, IPP Studies in the Frontiers of China's Public Policy,
https://doi.org/10.1007/978-981-99-6437-6_2

be translated into economic growth and social progress. In this international context, China was in the greatest crisis, which had involved in low growth rates, inefficient economic policies, and an increasing population. The domestic politics of the Cultural Revolution during 1966 and 1976 exaggerated the chaotic political situation. In 1966, Mao launched the Cultural Revolution, calling the Chinese young people to criticize party cadres who had betrayed the revolutionary spirit. During the 1970s, China also pursued a strategy of agricultural modernization, basic education improvement, and rural industrialization, which was known as "in agriculture, learning from Dazhai" (農業學大寨). The rural development strategy was implemented by the communes at the local level. The healthcare reform was precisely implemented in this context. This chapter identifies that the implementation of the barefoot doctor program as part of cooperative medical services (合作醫療), which changed the physician–patient relationship in rural areas in the late 1960s. Moving beyond a nostalgic view, this chapter explains that the key to understanding the well-functioning of the barefoot doctor program was the joint liability provided by the cooperative medical services.

2.1 Incorporating Chinese and Western Medicine into Villages

After its foundation in 1949, the Chinese Communist Party (hereinafter "CCP") government was committed to healthcare modernization in the context of state building. The quasi-constitutional Common Program (共同綱領) requires the state to assume the obligations to "promote mass sports, develop medical and health services, and protect health of mothers, infants, and children".[3] The Ministry of Health was also formally established in 1949, and after that, the Ministry of Health gradually expanded its organizational resources and functional differentiation. Despite the institutional establishment and expansion, the Ministry of Health was still highly constrained by financial resources. During the period from 1950 to 1957, the government health spending only accounted for 1.2%, while the national defense was 26.5%.[4] Although

[3] Quoted from Yanzhong Huang, *Governing Health in Contemporary China*, Milton Park, Abingdon, Oxon; New York: Routledge, 2013, p. 25.

[4] Huang, *Governing Health in Contemporary China*, p. 26.

the Ministry of Health was financially constrained, its responsibilities had been continuously increasing. The Government Insurance Scheme ((hereinafter "GIS") and the Labor Insurance Scheme ((hereinafter "LIS") were established, respectively, in 1951 and 1952, with the former covering government employees, college teachers, etc., and the former covering workers and their dependents in state-owned industrial enterprises. Given that the workers covered by the two schemes increased the demand for healthcare services also grew, which led to the consequence that although the Ministry of Health was financially restrained and it had to ensure to provide quality and efficient health services. For this reason, the Ministry of Health had to take efficient measures, while the measures were differently taken in the rural and urban areas.

In rural areas, a top-down healthcare reform and reorganization was carried out to form a two-tier state medical system, consisting of county hospitals and numerous township-level union clinics. The union clinics were established to provide medical services to villagers, following the principle of "one clinic per township".[5] The county union clinics also dispatched medical staff members to provide regular mobile medical to villagers, and thus villagers had convenient access to healthcare services at the union clinics. However, villagers had very limited access to county hospitals. This was because medical coordination only existed in township-level communities and seldom occurred between county hospitals and township-level union clinics during the 1950s and 1960s.[6] During the period between 1949 and 1955, the township union clinics were financed by the user-pay health system; while during the period between 1956 and 1978, the union clinics were gradually financed by medical collectives, and township hospitals were financed by the state. According to the Regulations for Organizing Union Clinics issued by the then Ministry of Health in 1956, "a union clinic was a socialist health and welfare entity under the ownership of a doctor's collective (醫生集體所有制) and established voluntarily by doctors under the leadership of the party and the government".[7] This suggests the emergence of a new form of health financing system.

[5] *See* Chapter One of Xiaoping Fang, *Barefoot Doctors and Western Medicine in China*, Rochester, NY: University of Rochester Press, 2012.

[6] Fang, *Barefoot Doctors and Western Medicine in China*, pp. 129–30.

[7] Ibid., 24.

The year 1968 marked the beginning of a massive public health initiative which had far-reaching effects in China. The centerpiece of the initiative was the implementation of the barefoot doctor program in rural China. Termed as "newly emerged things," barefoot doctors replaced the previous roles played by private physicians and folk healers in rural areas. Barefoot doctors presented a revolutionary image of young people, wading unexhausted through miles of rice paddies to provide healthcare services.[8] As members of the lowest level of the three-tiered state medical system comprising brigade health stations, commune clinics, and county hospitals, barefoot doctors participated in agricultural work as members of commune production brigades and simultaneously provided medical treatment and undertook public health work in their own production brigades.[9] Official media depicted barefoot doctors as Bethune, who were willing to work hard during morning and night and who were satisfied with receiving financial payment of the same amount as ordinary commune members. Although the latter might be simply a government propaganda, which exaggerated the obligation practices performed by barefoot doctors,[10] the improvement of the basic health care during 1949 and 1978 indicated its association with the barefoot doctor program and the Cooperative Medical System (hereinafter "CMS").[11] Sociological

[8] Judith Farquhar, "Market Magic: Getting Rich and Getting Personal in Medicine after Mao," *American Ethnologist* 23, 1996, p. 252.

[9] Fang, *Barefoot Doctors and Western Medicine in China*, p. 152.

[10] On December 8, 1968, an investigative report, "Cooperative medical service warmly welcomed by poor and lower-middle peasants," ("深受貧下中農歡迎的合作醫療制度") was published by the People's Daily, which introduced the cooperative medical service in Leyuan Commune, Hubei Province. It was also claimed by an official media that cooperative medical services and barefoot doctors were "great inventions made by poor and lower-middle peasants to combat diseases by depending on collective forces", and they "solved the problems of poor and lower-middle peasants seeking doctors, medicines, and health care". Termed as "newly emerged things", the national rollout of the barefoot doctor program was facilitated through large-scale media propaganda. Thirty-nine reports were published by the *People's Daily*, which had "cooperative medical service" in their titles during December 5, 1968 and December 21, 1969; and, thirty reports with the key words "barefoot doctors" in the titles were published by the *People's Daily* during September 14, 1968 and December 27, 1969. *See* Fang, *Barefoot Doctors and Western Medicine in China*, pp. 32–3 and note 88 on p. 217; *see* also Zhang, Wen & Liang, *From Barefoot Doctors to Village Doctors*.

[11] Peter Worsley notes that the World Health Assembly passed a resolution in1976 requesting that member states should take steps to promote the development of primary healthcare programs which included traditional medicine and curers. One of the primary

and anthropological research document barefoot doctors as hardworking, honest, and familiar with their fellow villagers; while villagers felt relaxed in their daily encounters and communication with their familiar barefoot doctors about their diseases, they also trusted barefoot doctors and deeply admired their spirit of sacrifice.[12] What are the obligation practices of barefoot doctors? What can their obligation practices reveal about the shifting nature of physician obligation and the bond between physicians and patients before and after the introduction of the barefoot program?

The barefoot doctor program was a crucial component of the state-driven medical modernization. Unlike the Nationalists claiming to provide "state medicine" for all, the CCP government claimed "to serve workers, peasants, and soldiers", but the healthcare institutional arrangements were made in favor of certain sections of the rural population.[13] In 1952, free GIS was granted to civil servants, party members, and disabled revolutionary veterans; LIS was also given to workers in state-owned enterprises.[14] Ordinary peasants, however, did not receive the public provision of healthcare services, except for infectious disease inoculation, sporadic free clinical services, and local disease treatment.[15] Realizing the large urban–rural inequalities in the healthcare system, in 1965 Mao harshly criticized the situation:

> [t]he Ministry of Health is only able to serve 15 percent of the total population, and this 15 percent is made up mostly of the privileged. The broad ranks of the peasants cannot obtain medical treatment and also do

stimuli for the World Health Assembly to promote this was the publicity given in the Western countries to Chinese acupuncture, the traditional pharmacopoeia, and the primary healthcare system based on barefoot doctors. *See* Peter Worsley, "Non-Western Medical Systems," *Annual Review of Anthropology* 11(1), 1982, p. 340; *see* also World Health Organization and the United Nations Children's Fund, "Primary Health Care: A Joint Report by the Director-General of the World Health Organization and the Executive Director of the United Nations Children's Fund," International Conference on Primary Health Care, Alma-Ata, USSR, September 1978.

12 *See* for instance Sydney D. White "From 'Barefoot Doctor' to 'Village Doctor' in Tiger Springs Village: A Case Study of Rural Health Care Transformations in Socialist China," *Human Organization* 57(4), 1998, pp. 480–90; *see* also Zhang, Wen & Liang, *From Barefoot Doctors to Village Doctors*.

13 Fang, *Barefoot Doctors and Western Medicine in China*, p. 29.

14 Ibid.

15 Ibid.

> not receive medicine. The Ministry of Health is not a people's ministry. It should be called the Urban Health Ministry, the Ministry of Health for the Lords, or even the Urban Ministry of Health for the Lords ... Stress rural areas in medial and heath work![16]

This statement later became the famous "June 26 Directive". In response to Mao's call to focus health care in rural areas, the national rollout of the barefoot doctor program started in the late 1960s. The selection, training, and behaviors of barefoot doctors were all under rigorous ideological indoctrination and political control which were commonplace during the era of the Cultural Revolution. Basic knowledge of Western and Chinese traditional medicine was conveyed to them through the reference books—such as *Barefoot Doctor's Manual*—and periodic training sessions.[17]

Political dominance was then omnipresent. The medical ethics for barefoot doctors assumed a political meaning under the socialist system. During the 1970s, barefoot doctors were required by the medical ethics to be both "red and expert", "meaning socialist in spirit and medically proficient".[18] The image of barefoot doctors was expected to exemplify "the New Man of Chinese Socialism" to give expression to the spirit of collectivism and service.[19] After 1970, a series of awards was further introduced to reinforce the public recognition of outstanding doctors and strengthen the sense of group identity and doctors' obligations. For instance, "'model barefoot doctors' were celebrated at representative meetings, which also involved group political training of the barefoot doctors to further encourage the formation of an *esprit de corps* and a united idea of medical ethics".[20]

The good performance of barefoot doctors was also inseparable from a strict system of monitoring and control. "At that time, barefoot doctors were studying very hard, and there was a meeting every half a month,

[16] Quoted from ibid., p 30.

[17] *See* Sydney White, "From 'Barefoot Doctor' to 'Village Doctor' in Tiger Springs Village: A Case Study of Rural Health Care Transformations in Socialist China," *Human Organization* 57 (1998), p. 482.

[18] Ibid., 157.

[19] Judith Farquhar, "Market Magic: Getting Rich and Getting Personal in Medicine after Mao," *American Ethnologist* 23(2), 1996, p. 242.

[20] Fang, *Barefoot Doctors and Western Medicine in China*, 157.

so as to convey the work requirements of his superiors and implement disease prevention tasks. [Thus], [c]ooperative medical care was a set of systems, a system, and barefoot doctors were part of this system, which played the role under the management of the system".[21] The monitoring and control of healthcare service provision was mainly implemented through inspecting barefoot doctors' "prescriptions". All prescriptions issued by barefoot doctors were retained and selected for inspection by the commune health center and the cooperative medical management committee. All registration fees (5 cents per prescription) were handed over to the commune health center at the regular meeting, which were also checked with the prescriptions.[22]

Moreover, the trust between barefoot doctors and villagers was developed through continuous interactions. Barefoot doctors replaced the previous roles played by folk healers in rural China. Before the advent of barefoot doctors, China's rural medical landscape had been dominated by folk healers, while professional physicians were only a minority.[23] Only elites had access to the healthcare services provided by physicians. Folk healers and patients were embedded in close relations of the same enclosed communities. Patients and their family members were allowed to engage in the healing process.[24] The CCP government improved the health care of ordinary people and seemed willing to work with local groups and individuals in a united front to facilitate socialist progress. This attempt won support from home and abroad. Chen Zhiqian recalled that "As a physician with strong patriotic feelings, I looked forward to contribute to health improvement in the new socialist society".[25] In other words, CCP's attempts at engaging with the masses in public health were a core part of its socialistic transformative project, as an alternative model of public health.

[21] Zhang, Wen & Liang, *From Barefoot Doctors to Village Doctors*, p. 49; *see* also Nianqun Yang, *Remaking the "Patient": The Politics of Space in the Conflict between Chinese and Western Medicine 1832–1985* [再造 "病人": 中西醫衝突下的空間政治] Beijing: Beijing Renmin University Press, p. 537.

[22] Yang, *Remaking the "Patient"*, p. 537.

[23] Fang, *Barefoot Doctors and Western Medicine in China*, p. 21.

[24] Ibid., 163.

[25] C.C. Chen, *Medicine in Rural China: A Personal Account*, Berkeley, Los Angeles, London: University of California Press, p. 119.

The advent of barefoot doctors not only facilitated the penetration of Western modern medical instruments and pharmaceuticals down into villages, but also increased the control of the barefoot doctors over the treatment processes and increased their authority in interactions with patients. For instance, the presence of a stethoscope shifted the power of judging illness from the hands of patients to those of barefoot doctors. Villagers were astonished to find that barefoot doctors were able to learn about the human body's structure through a stethoscope.[26] While the position and authority of barefoot doctors were ascended in the relations with patients, villagers' initial faith and trust were limited in barefoot doctors. After all, they only received a few months of training. A barefoot doctor described his experience by saying that:

> When I had just become a barefoot doctor in the village, the son of a peasant developed a high fever. When I heard this news, I went to his home without being asked. But his father insisted that the fever was due to mischief caused by ghosts and gods. He set up a shrine and burned spirit paper, and then he mixed the ashes with water and asked his son to drink this mixture. However, his child's fever became more and more serious.[27]

As the illness became more serious, the child's father allowed the barefoot doctor to treat his son's fever. It turned out that the child's common cold had developed into pneumonia. The child's temperature finally dropped after doses of herbal medicine. As said by the barefoot doctor, "[a]fter this event, the people living in nearby villages were willing to ask me to treat them".[28] This suggests that while the ideological indoctrination and political control were effectively implemented, the trust between barefoot doctors and village patients was not necessarily developed by them. Rather, the trust and respect were gradually developed through their continuous, real, and sympathetic interactions.

[26] Stanley Joel Reiser, *Technological Medicine: The Changing World of Doctors and Patients*, New York: Cambridge University Press, 2009, pp. 7–8.

[27] Fang, *Barefoot Doctors and Western Medicine in China*, p. 164.

[28] Ibid.

2.2 Decommodification of Healthcare

The non-profit orientation of the collective medical services was also essential to the practice of medicine under the barefoot doctor program. The collective medical services were a rural form of healthcare insurance, while the operation of the barefoot doctor program was supported by the CMS. During 1969 and 1977, the CMS was widely adopted, which guaranteed the operation of the barefoot doctor program. Under the CMS, the non-profit orientation of the barefoot doctor program could be observed in two respects. Healthcare services and medicine were not deemed as commodities to be produced for sale; rather, most medical expenses were shared by collectives and their members via the operation of the CMS. The typical characteristics of the CMS were characterized as follows:

> First, the CMS expenses were shared by collectives (public welfare funds) as well as individuals (fees). Second, cooperative medical services were not legally mandatory, but in communes and brigades that adopted the system, participation was compulsory and user fees were deducted by the collectives before income distribution at the end of the year. Third, cooperative medical services relied on low-cost barefoot doctors who helped reduce medical costs to an affordable level by raising herbs and making Chinese herbal medicine on their own.[29]

Given that the Chinese government did not impose a nationwide model of the CMS, the CMS varied across brigades, communes, counties, and regions. The proportion of the collective contribution to the medical funds also differed, ranging from 30 to 90% of the collective funds. In most localities, peasants had to pay a small amount of registration fee, ranging from 1 to 3 *yuan* for each person and each year. The registration fees were usually reduced directly from the collective fund before peasants' compensations were allocated.[30] From the standpoint of peasants, after paying the registration fees, they could receive healthcare services without any additional costs. Thus, peasants did not view the healthcare services and medicines as commodities produced for sale; they also trusted

[29] Shaoguang Wang, "Adapting by Learning: The Evolution of China's Rural Health Care Financing," *Modern China* 35, 2009, pp. 380–1.

[30] Ibid., 381.

that barefoot doctors could provide truly affordable and accessible healthcare services. This further ensured that peasants would not lose faith in and respect for barefoot doctors due to unaffordable healthcare expenses.

Compensations received by barefoot doctors were in the form of work points. Like their fellow villagers, the daily work of each barefoot doctor was decided by his or her physical capacity for undertaking agricultural work, while medical qualifications, proficiency, and the number of patients that barefoot doctors treated did not affect their compensations.[31] The compensation calculation methods also minimized internal competition and conflicts. For instance, Shengju Yan was a barefoot doctor at Longzhang Brigade medical service station. He was the third barefoot doctor of the medical service station. According to him, all the three barefoot doctors received work points for thirty days every month, but there were discrepancies among them. Like other normal laborers, Yan received 10 work points. Another elder barefoot doctor received 8.5 points due to his old age, while a female barefoot doctor only received 6 points due to her female gender.[32] Barefoot doctors accepted the calculation methods of the work point system.[33] The compensation methods and discrepancies in earnings did not create incentives for them to provide more services. Thus, the non-profit orientation of the healthcare services provided by barefoot doctors was also a crucial factor in ensuring that unnecessary healthcare services would not be produced by them.

While the national rollout of barefoot doctors in rural China marked the beginning the state-driven medical modernization and the introduction of Western medicine started to increase their authority in interactions with patients, the non-profit orientation of healthcare services under the collective medical services added an atmosphere of deep trust between barefoot doctors and village patients. The decommodification of medicine and healthcare characterizes "a communal responsibility".[34] The distribution of medicine and health care is solely based on needs rather than patients' abilities to pay. The collective assumes the primary obligation to

[31] Fang, *Barefoot Doctors and Western Medicine in China*, p. 155.

[32] Ibid.

[33] Ibid., 157.

[34] Cong, "Doctor-Family-Patient Relationship," p. 164. It is noted by Cong that between 1949 and 1978, "socialist communism was the basic principle in the field of general ethics, including medical ethics". One of the salient characteristics of such a health system was the sacrifice of the interests of individuals to those of the community.

finance the public healthcare system in the rural areas, while the state did not assume the obligation, needless to say legal obligation to finance it.[35]

The funding of the barefoot doctor program can be better observed against the wider background of nation building in China, especially when compared with other publicly supported health systems, such as the NHS in the United Kingdom (hereinafter "UK"). In the UK, the NHS was created out of the idea that "healthcare should not be viewed as a commodity—that is, as something produced for sale on a market".[36] Out of this consideration, the health care was made available "without charge", which thereby removed the element of profit from health care. The decommodification of health care in the UK was consistent with that of the cooperative medical system in China. However, different from the cooperative medical system in China, the NHS was funded by general taxation, which reflected that "this mode of financing the NHS involve[d] an element of redistribution in the form of providing a healthcare service for all citizens irrespective of means, it [could] also be considered to reflect principles similar to those underpinning the old Roman Law notion of *obligatio in solidum*—namely, that each member of a group 'is liable for the reversal of fortunes of another'".[37] The taxation was therefore not simply a means of funding revenue for healthcare, but a "socio-financial democratic contract" which established the linkage "between mass taxation and social rights".[38]

In contrast with the mode of funding for health care, the cooperative medical services in China were not financially supported by general taxation, or any taxation mechanism, but by the public welfare funds of the commune in villages as well as fees paid by individual villagers. The particular mode of financing suggests that the cooperative medical system at most involved the redistribution and solidarity in the form of providing

[35] In the UK, the institution of the NHS was characterized as "a communal responsibility". According to the first Act of 1946, it is the duty of the Minister of Health to promote the establishment of the institution designed to improve the physical and mental health of the people in England and Wales, and the health services "shall be free of charge". The free and equal provision of health services is therefore characterized as a communal responsibility.

[36] Kenneth Veitch, "Obligation and the Changing Nature of Publicly Funded Healthcare," *Medical Law Review* 27(2), 2019, p. 272.

[37] Ibid., 273.

[38] Ibid., 274.

a healthcare service for all villagers in the same commune or town, rather than all citizens irrespective of means. If the cooperative medical system was put against the wider background of nation building, it was not established.

Thus, this chapter identifies that the source of the sense of obligation of barefoot doctors was to be found in their real and sympathetic interactions with fellow villagers. The proximity of the relationship between barefoot doctors and fellow villagers in the tightly knit community of villages provided them with constant interactions and the opportunity for respect and trust to endure. The institutionalized political control and the decommodification of the healthcare services under the CMS were also identified as important factors that could not be separated from barefoot doctors' discharge of obligations. The decommodification of healthcare services and the collective nature of the CMS were crucial in shaping the obligation practices of barefoot doctors and their patients. This analysis matters as it is precisely the decommodification of healthcare services and medicine that is reasserting our memories of barefoot doctors and the CMS. With the historical dimensions and the source of ethical sense of obligation of barefoot doctors, it can be better understood why the economic reform in 1978 may fundamentally change the obligations underpinning the bond of trust between physicians and patients, which will be identified and discussed in the following chapters. As the state continued to play the leading role in transforming the Chinese medical system after 1970s, the barefoot doctor program gradually faded away and pharmaceuticals and medical services became products being sold in the market. How the medical reform since 1978 changed the obligations underpinning the bond of trust between physicians and patients will be identified and discussed in the following chapters.

CHAPTER 3

Incorporation of Western Bioethics into China

During the period between 1911 and 1949, the principle "penetrat[ing] into all the medical professions and form[ing] the basis of the socialist principles of medical ethics" was the ethical mandate promulgated by Mao Zedong, "[r]escue the dying, heal the wounded, and execute revolutionary humanism" (救死扶傷, 實行革命的人道主義).[1] This principle was written by Chairman Mao for the China Medical University in May 1941.[2] The medical principle suggests that physicians should satisfy the interests of patients without considering their personal interests. The obligations of doctors were ethical in the sense that they were derived from the ethical principles of medicine and health care. Since 1949, socialist communism has been the basic principle in the field of "general ethics", including medical ethics.[3] Communism suggests that the consistency of the interests of the community and those of the individual, which can be expressed by the saying that "[t]he aim of people's behavior is the interests of the community; only if the community's interests can be met, can

[1] H. Zhang, Z. He & L. Chi, *A Survey of Chinese Foreign Medical Moral Standards*, Tianjin: Tianjin Ancient Books Press, 2000, p. 385; quoted from Cong, "Doctor-Family-Patient Relationship," p. 163.

[2] Cong, "Doctor-Family-Patient Relationship," p. 163.

[3] Ibid., 164.

L. Jia, *Obligation*, IPP Studies in the Frontiers of China's Public Policy,
https://doi.org/10.1007/978-981-99-6437-6_3

the individual's interests be sought".[4] Since 1952, under the influence of the "Learn from Soviet Union" movement, Soviet medicine with a typical representative of the Pavlovian theory was adopted as "dialectically materialistic".[5] The Soviet model of medicine based on protectiveness was institutionalized in China, which argues that "[i]t is the duty of health care professionals to mobilize all the strengths of the patient against his or her disease and to develop this attitude of strength in the patient".[6] This is because the ideology of protectiveness believes that the psychological relationship of the patient to the disease occupies a central position in the healing process.[7] In addition, during this period the communist socialist system enabled everyone to have an equal access to free medical care. It means that when patients could not afford to pay hospitals and physicians would also treat them without discrimination.[8] Thus, under the influence of socialist communism as well as the Soviet model of medicine, the traditional paternalist relationship between physicians and patients was added by the emergence of "deep trust in the doctor".[9]

The preceding changes of the physician–patient relationship demonstrate different features. Against the wider backdrop of establishing the publicly funded healthcare system, the traditional paternalist physician–patient relationship was changed into decision-making between family members and physicians although patient autonomy was not fully achieved.[10] According to a renowned Chinese medical ethicist, Cong Yali, "If we say that phase one's style of DPR [doctor-patient relationship] was still traditional paternalism, then phase two strengthened it by adding an atmosphere of deep trust in the doctor".[11] One of the most important reasons for the formation of the deep trust between patients

[4] Y. Wei, *New Ethics Teaching*, Beijing: Beijing University Press, 2000, p. 310, quoted from ibid.

[5] Qiu Renzong, "Philosophy of Medicine in China (1939–1980)," *Theoretical Medicine and Bioethics* 3(1), 1982, p. 37.

[6] Mei-che Samantha Pang, "Protective Truthfulness: The Chinese Way of Safeguarding Patients in Informed Treatment Decisions," *Journal of Medical Ethics* 25, 1999, p. 249.

[7] Ibid.

[8] Cong, "Doctor-Family-Patient Relationship," p. 164.

[9] Ibid.

[10] Ibid., 163.

[11] Ibid., 164.

and doctors was the healthcare system. The socialist healthcare system, as also sketched above, allowed "almost every person [to] enjoy equal and free medical care". Even for those who could not afford the medical costs (patients needed to pay the costs before getting a refund from work units), Cong said, "the hospital and the doctor would also treat him without difference".[12] Given that the health care was received free of charge, doctors did not have any individual interests in profit-making in the socialist healthcare system during this period, which Cong believes prevented the potential of arising interest conflicts between patients and doctors.[13] In this sense, compared with the social relationship between physicians and patients in the first phase, the second phase demonstrated a strengthened paternalist relationship between physicians and patients. Thus, the relationship was changed due to the formation of the socialist healthcare system, which is a structural reason, and it was also affected by the principle of medical ethics.

As noted above, the publicly funded health care during the Mao period of China saw the improvement of people's health conditions. The social bond between citizens and the state was also created during this period especially in the urban areas. The late 1970s, however, witnessed a series of healthcare reforms that were proposed along with the shift of the overall agenda from a planned economy toward economic development. If the 1960s and 1970s witnessed the incorporation of the Chinese and Western medicine into rural China, the 1980s further saw Western modernization and liberal ideas penetrating into Chinese medicine and health care. This chapter explains the incorporation of two important Western medical ethics—the doctrine of informed consent and the right to health—and how they have been conciliated with the Chinese medicine and healthcare institutions. To highlight the introduction of the doctrine of informed consent is to explain the changing practices of physician and patient obligations to disclose related information to patients and their family members; while to discuss the different views of the right to health is to further analyze the role and function of state in the particular context of modernization and healthcare provision in contemporary China.

[12] Ibid.

[13] Ibid.

3.1 Doctrine of Informed Consent

At a time when the relations between physicians and patients were no longer personal ones, nor even one-to-one relationship, but rather between patients and organizations staffed by medical professionals, the nature of the physician–patient relationship might be different from the one between barefoot doctors and their patients. This section identifies and discusses the obligations of physicians and patients and the bond of trust between them in the context of marketization of health care during 1978–2002. The analysis concerns how the ethical doctrine of informed consent was incorporated into the Chinese medical context.

Since the early 1980s, a series of textbooks and monographs of medical ethics were published by the first generation scholars in China, including Professor Qiu Renzong, He Zhaoxiong, Du Zhizheng, Li Benfu, Shi Dapu, and Pen Ruicong. After the Cultural Revolution, the first textbook of bioethics was published by Zhizheng Du in 1985. In 1987, Renzong Qiu published *Bioethics*, which was the first textbook that systemically introduced Western bioethics into China. In 1988, Zhaoxiong He published *History of Chinese Medical Morality* (Table 3.1).

The doctrine of informed consent initially appeared in scholars' translated works, textbooks, and academic conferences before it was incorporated into the Chinese law. In 1985, *Introduction to Medical Ethics* (醫

Table 3.1 The textbook, monographs, and translated works (1980s–2010s)

Author	*Name of textbooks, monographs, and translated works*	*Year*
Zhizheng Du	Outlines of Medical Ethics	1985
Renzong Qiu	Bioethics	1987
Zhaoxiong He	History of Medical Morality	1988
Benfu LI	Textbook of Medical Ethics	1996
Hongzhu Zhang	Survey of Chinese and Foreign Medical Moral Standards	2000
Singer, translated by Shen Liu	Practical Ethics	1995
H. Tristram Engelhardt, Jr., Ruiping Fan	Foundation of Bioethics	2006
Translated by Jingbao Nie and Linying Hu	Classic Cases in Medical Ethics	2010
Translated by Xia Lin	Intervention and Reflection: Basic Issues in Medical Ethics	2010

學倫理學概論) edited by He Zhaoxiong was published, which marked the beginning of ethical analysis of specific issues in medical development and clinical medical work, and bioethics. Drawing upon the development of medical ethics in the United States, he highlighted that the doctrine of informed consent reflected the value of patent autonomy and explained that the right to informed consent as a kind of patient rights contained the right to accept and refuse to accept medical interventions.[14] In 1987, the book, *Bioethics* written by Qiu Renzong was published by Shanghai People's Publishing House, which established the theoretical framework of Chinese bioethics. Qiu Renzong further elaborated the legal doctrine of informed consent in *Patients' Rights*, which specified the four core elements of informed consent, i.e., the standards for information disclosure, requirements for full understanding of patients, standards for voluntary consent, and the capacity for understanding.[15] The introduction of the doctrine of informed consent paved the way for the legal incorporation of such a doctrine.

The doctrine of informed consent was not mandated by a statutory requirement in Chinese until the 1980s, including Art 40 of the 1982 Regulation on Medical Work,[16] Art 33 of 1994 Regulation on the Administration of Medical Institutions,[17] Art 62 of the Detailed Rules on the Implementation of Regulation on the Administration of Medical

[14] Zhaoxiong He & Lixing Chen, eds. *Introduction to Medical Ethics* [醫學倫理學概論], Nanjing: Jiangsu Science and Technology Publishing House, 1985, pp. 30, 39.

[15] Renzong Qiu & Jianmei Feng, *Patients' Rights* [病人的權利], Beijing: Medical University and Peking Union Medical College, 1996, pp. 58–64.

[16] Art 40.6 of Regulation on Medical Work (1982, Ministry of Health) (醫院工作制度) stipulates that before the operation of a surgery, consent in writing must be sought from family members or work units of the patient (excerpt for surface surgery). When the emergency operation is too late to seek the consent from the family members or units, it can be signed by the attending physician and approved by the director of the department, the dean or the deputy dean of the operation.

[17] Art 33 of Regulation on Medical Institution (1994, State Council) (醫療機構管理條例) stipulates that "when administering 'operations, special examination, or special treatment,' the medical institution should obtain the consent of the patient and his or her family members or relatives".

Institutions enacted in 1994,[18] Art 26 of the Law on Medical Practitioners enacted in 1998,[19] and Art 11 of 2002 Regulation on Handling of Medical Accidents.[20] Pursuant to these regulations, physicians are obligated to truthfully inform patients or their family members of the patient's conditions without incurring adverse impacts on the patients. In other words, both patients and their family members are entitled to be informed and to consent. Before the promulgation of 2009 Tort Liability Law, these legislations were only subject to a breach of the obligation of informed consent to disciplinary and administrative punishments. While these legislations specify the legal obligations to protect the right to informed consent, when the notion of informed consent was first introduced to the China's healthcare context it was not so central to the physician–patient relations, which were dominated by a paternalist view. Given that informed consent was originally a Western moral concept, it was considered as incompatible with Chinese cultural tradition and inapplicable to the healthcare context of China for a long time. This subsection explores the discussions on the applicability of informed consent to the healthcare context of China and draws out some key themes concerning the obligations of physicians and patients.

Turning first to Nie's article, he questions the "culture differences" argument against the applicability of informed consent in China—namely, that informed consent, as a Western moral concept representing the notion of individualism, is fundamentally incompatible with the communitarian Confucian orientation of Chinese culture. In doing this, the author proposes a two-part argument. The first part suggests that to emphasize the fundamental differences between Western and Chinese cultures not only fails to appreciate the integration of the diverse value

[18] Art 62 of Rules for Implementing the Regulation on Medical Institutions (1994, Ministry of Health) (醫療機構管理條例實施細則) specifies that "the medical institution should respect the patient's right to be informed of his condition, diagnosis and treatment, and, when administrating operations, special examination and special treatment, the medical institution should give the patient 'necessary explanations'".

[19] Art 26 of Law on Practicing Doctors of the People's Republic of China (1998) (中華人民共和國執業醫師法) stipulates that "doctors should truthfully explain the patients' condition to the patients or their family members".

[20] Art 11 of Regulation on the Handling of Medical Accidents (2002, State Council) (醫療事故處理條例) provides that "when providing medical treatment, medical institutions and medical practitioners should truthfully inform patients of their condition, treatment measures, medical risks and other information".

systems, but misconstrues the real issue at stake. As argued by Nie, at the heart of the matter is the power relations between patients and physicians as well as medical institutions. The second part tries to justify the compatibility between the doctrine of informed consent and Chinese culture. To do this, Nie argues that the doctrine of informed consent can be justified from both individualist and communitarian perspectives, while Chinese culture is also a combination of both communitarian and individualist traditions.

The author's critique begins with an observation that informed consent is probably the most important concept in contemporary bioethics not only as an academic discipline but as a socio-cultural movement, which has significantly contributed to the historical change of medical ethics from a professionalized, physician-centered, and paternalist mode to a patient-centered one in the Western context. Arguing that informed consent is based on Western individualism, in particular the notion of individual autonomy, while Chinese culture is based on communitarian Confucianism, which is fundamentally incommensurable with the Western one, Nie comments: "according to this argument, informed consent is defined primarily as an issue of culture. However, in reality it is mainly concerned with the issue of power".[21] Nie's argument is that informed consent helps to empower patients and prevent the power abuse by physicians, and in the context of health care, the unbalanced power at stake is the physicians' professional power brought by their medical expertise and knowledge. To recognize the right to informed consent is to enable patients to jointly participate in the decision-making related to health care and thereby be free from "force, fraud, deceit, duress, overreaching, or other ulterior forms of constraint or coercion".[22] Just as in Western countries, there are unequal power relations between physicians and patients in China. To endow patients the right to informed consent is therefore to empower patients via joint participation in the decision-making.[23]

Nie also proposes that despite that informed consent is always given an expression by individual rights and justified by reference to individual

[21] Nie, *Medical Ethics in China*, p. 136.

[22] The Nuremberg Code identifies four essential elements of "valid consent"—namely, "it must be voluntary (i.e. free from 'force, fraud, deceit, duress, overreaching, or other ulterior forms of constraint or coercion'), legally valid, informed, and fully comprehended by the subject)". Quoted from ibid., 134.

[23] Ibid., 136.

autonomy it is also a matter of the common good. By reference to Joseph Raz's influential communitarian justification for rights, Nie clarifies that a right that ultimately benefits an individual has communal, or in Nie's words communitarian aspects. As put by Raz, "rights by definition mean to hold someone or certain authorities to be under a duty so that rights and duties are correlative and never separable".[24] What is suggested by Raz is that rights not simply have individualist aspects in the sense that it is individuals who ultimately benefit from the participation in rights, but also have communal aspects in the sense that rights impose multiple kinds of—rather than a single kind of—correlative duties on a number of duty bearers. In light of this, to secure the right to informed consent relies on the performance of multiple kinds of duties by various duty bearers and dischargers, in particular physicians.

Informed consent has a communal aspect in respect of promoting the bond of mutual trust between physicians and patients. The bond of mutual trust is an essential communal aspect of the doctrine of informed consent. By reference to Annette Baier's prominent article, trust is understood as "reliance on others' competence and willingness to look after, rather than harm, things one cares about".[25] The bond of trust between physicians and patients is established upon patients' reliance on physicians' knowledge, expertise, and willingness to provide medical services. Nie further notes that the bond of trust is a fragile one in that the interests of patients may be overridden by physicians, while this is inevitable because it is precisely due to the power and knowledge imbalances between physicians and patients that the trust can be established.[26] As said by Richard Holton, "When you trust someone to do something, you rely on them to do it, and you regard that reliance in a certain way: you have a readiness to feel betrayal should it be disappointed, and gratitude should it be upheld".[27] In this sense, what matters is to ensure that the interests of patients are not easily overridden by physicians. In Baier's analysis, to strive to achieve the equalizing power, rather than simply exercise the

[24] Ibid., 140–1.

[25] Annette Baier, "Trust and Antitrust," *Ethics* 96(2), 1986, p. 234.

[26] Jing-Bao Nie, Lun Li, Grant Gillett, Joseph D. Tucker & Arthur Kleinman, "The Crisis of Patient-Physician Trust and Bioethics: Lessons and Inspirations from China," *Developing World Bioethics* 18, 2017, p. 64.

[27] Richard Holton, "Deciding to Trust, Coming to Believe," *Australasian Journal of Philosophy* 72, 1994, p. 67.

power of superior medical understanding, is the key to achieving a trustworthy attitude. Baier says, "trust is appropriately placed in those who, for whatever motives, welcome the equalization of power, who assist the less powerful and renounce eminence of power, who, when they ask us to delay the accounting of their use of discretionary power, do so for reasons that we will eventually see to have been good (as good parents correctly tell their young children 'one day you will understand, but not yet. And it is so that you will one day understand, and be my equal, that I ask you now to trust me')".[28] The doctrine of informed consent is precisely the tool which can prevent patients' views from being paternalistically overridden and which enables their views to be better heard, respected, and protected. To achieve this, physicians must act upon the obligations as required by the notion of informed consent. Thus, as put by Nie, "[i]nformed consent can be viewed as the best way of promoting trust between patients (the public) and physicians (the medical profession)".[29] Nie's analysis of family consent also recognizes the significance of patients' joint participation in the decision-making by noting that the real danger of paternalism is not simply that family members may deny necessary medical treatments for patients, and patients' privacy may not be appropriately protected, but also that "the judgments made by family members about the best interests may not accord to the genuine best interests in the views of patients themselves".[30] In the healthcare context of China, however, the bond of trust between physicians and patients was an extremely fragile and deteriorating one, considering an increasing number of violence and murders against medical professionals.[31] To restore the bond of trust between physicians and patients, Nie suggests that several measures should be taken, including not simply that the communication skills as demanded by the doctrine of informed consent should be improved, but that social policies ought to be formulated to reform the current healthcare system and to better protect patients' rights.

Nie's article, which offers a convincing argument for the compatibility of informed consent with Chinese cultures, has been picked up from

[28] Annette Baier, *Moral Prejudices: Essays on Ethics*, Cambridge: Harvard University Press, 1994, pp. 180–1.

[29] Nie, *Medical Ethics in China*, p. 141.

[30] Ibid., 144.

[31] Ibid., 141.

legal perspectives. Vera Lúcia Raposo engages in a discussion of family informed consent.[32] The core theme concerned is whether, and under which circumstances, the Chinese law should impose informed consent for medical treatments on patients or their family members. As well as proposing that a set of legal obligations and liabilities should be imposed on physicians to disclose the information related to medical treatments and to seek consent from patients and their family members except for emergency situations, Raposo argues that the informed consent of individual patients should be adopted due to its compatibility with human rights. In the Western context, legal discussions also revolve around patient obligations correlative to the right to informed consent. For instance, as argued by Draper and Sorell, the notion of informed consent not only denotes a genuine partnership between physicians and patients in medical treatment, but the "joint responsibility for the outcomes".[33] In the sense that "[a]utonomy without responsibility is not autonomy, even where the autonomy is a vulnerable patient's autonomy", obligations are also incumbent on patients.[34]

The above articles, and the arguments in them, have three implicit key themes which concern our discussion of the obligations underpinning the bonds between physicians and patients. First, Nie's and Raposo's articles offer normative inquiries into what should be done to empower patients through information disclosure. Their arguments concern the particular kinds of obligation ought to be discharged and the manner in which obligations should be done by physicians to respect patients' right to be informed and to consent; in particular, they engage with the question of what particular kind of information ought to be disclosed by physicians. Their discussions reveal that the decisions ought to be in the best interests of the patients, but also demands that the responsibility for the outcomes of the joint decisions also ought to be shared by them.[35] These ethical requirements denote that not any kind of decisions can be made, and that there ought to be a genuine partnership and trust between physicians and patients in the sense of sharing the liabilities incurred by the decisions.

[32] Vera Lúcia Raposo, "Lost in 'Culturation': Medical Informed Consent in China (from a Western Perspective)," *Medicine, Health Care and Philosophy* 22, 2019.

[33] Heather Draper & Tom Sorell, "Patients' Responsibilities in Medical Ethics," *Bioethics* 16(4), 2002, pp. 339–40.

[34] Ibid., 340.

[35] *See* Ibid.

Second, let me turn to the correlative point, namely that the right to informed consent does not generate a single form of obligation. Jeremy Waldron, drawing on the work of Joseph Raz, argues that when rights are considered, a right generates what is called by Waldron "waves of duties", which questions the equal and one-to-one standing between rights and duties. One reading of Waldron's point is that a right may generate duties to be performed by many people. Yet what Waldron suggests is more than this. As put by Scott Veitch, what Waldron argues is that "we cannot fully understand the operation of this right in practice unless we see that the same right generates not just one duty of this sort, but of multiple ***kinds*** of duties (hence the 'waves' image)".[36] The "waves of duties" account is not simply one corresponding to our understanding about the multiple forms of legal obligations arising from a legal right, but a normative inquiry into how best to protect the legal right if the legal right is to be taken seriously.

The above two points are linked. This is in particular so as regards Nie's argument which extends beyond the correlativity of the right and obligations to the ethical senses of physician obligation—the other-regarding aspect that points to the central characteristic of obligation—the idea of the bond between physicians and patients. This can be observed, for instance, from Nie's argument that "[i]nformed consent can be viewed as the best way of promoting trust between patients (the public) and physicians (the medical profession)".[37] Drawing on the theories of philosopher Annette Baier and legal scholar Mark Henaghan, in Nie's approach to trust and informed consent, trust emerges where patients are empowered by the right to informed consent. When this is so, there arises equal footing between physicians and patients: to meet the ethical requirements for physicians to protect patients' right to informed consent requires that patients should be well informed and fully understand what is proposed, and they thus should be placed in a position to choose or refuse in light of the information and understanding. Using Baier's analysis, "the most trustworthy attitude is to strive to equalise power as best as one can, regardless of the circumstances, rather than simply exercising power over

[36] Scott Veitch, "The Sense of Obligation," *Jurisprudence* 8(3), 2017, p. 420.

[37] Nie, *Medical Ethics in China*, p. 141.

another".[38] In the context of health care, while physicians have superior medical knowledge and expertise, they can demonstrate the attitude of equal power by good communication and knowledge sharing with patients, thereby fostering trust between physicians and patients. The performance of the physician obligations, including the ones correlative to the right to informed consent, therefore, can be viewed as a necessary condition for the sustenance of trust between physicians and patients.

But, as also indicated by Nie's reference to the severe and deteriorating physician–patient relationship, the ethical senses of physician obligation have not effectively existed in China. During 1978 and 2003, there arose an increasing number of conflicts between physicians and patients. In 2001 alone, there were over 500 violence cases of patients and patient members harming physicians.[39] The emergence of the large numbers of violence cases was a crisis of trust between physicians and patients, while behind the crisis laid very complicated economic conflicts of interest.[40] Despite this, Nie also notes that "[t]he illness journey in any place including China can be characterized as an extended locus of trust: intelligent listening and concern, careful diagnosis, conscientious treatment, responsive attention to the contingencies of a regimen of care, and non-abandonment are a sine qua non of ethical medicine and form a solid relational foundation for trust and trustworthiness".[41] What Nie suggests here is a new version of physician–patient interaction, which demands more than simply the change of attitudes of both physicians and patients, but changes in the conditions of medical practice; trust will reasonably thrive from where the changes of physician–patient interaction are achieved. Although trust itself is not directly related to explicit obligations, the trust between physicians and patients emerges from where there is equal footing between them by and through meeting the ethical obligations for physicians to protect patients' right to informed consent and meeting those for patients to understand and make a choice between healthcare service options in light of the understanding.

[38] Mark Henaghan, *Health Professionals and Trust: The Cure for Healthcare Law and Policy*, London: Routledge-Cvendish, 2011, p. 24.

[39] Cong, "Doctor, Family, Patient Relationship," p. 167.

[40] Ibid.

[41] Nie et al., "The Crisis of Patient-Physician Trust and Bioethics," pp. 1–9.

Third, the implementation of the right to informed consent in China also concerns the change of paternalist relationship between physicians and patients as well as their family members. The traditional relationship between physicians and patients as well as their family members was guided by Confucian cultures. This relationship was best characterized in the way that "a family member functions as a bridge between the patient and the doctor".[42] In this relationship, family members, usually the leader of a big family played the role of making decisions for the patient on behalf of the interests of the whole big family, while patients usually showed obedience to the authority of doctors. For Nie, family played crucial roles as a social institution and it was morally important in different societies and cultures. This was so in both Chinese and Western societies and cultures, which was shown by many cross-cultural empirical studies and observations. The real issue at stake about the roles of family in the healthcare context of China, however, was not a cultural concern but an economic one. The reason for physicians and hospitals to seek consent from family members rather than simply individual patients was to secure the payment of medical expenses and to reduce the risks of incurring medical malpractice liabilities against them.[43] The medical decisions made on the basis of family consent for the individual patient can thus be aligned with the best interests, including economic interests, of the family, rather than with the obligation to consider the true best interests of the patient's health. This reflects the real danger of family consent and paternalism in general. The implementation of informed consent in this sense is to avoid this danger.

The above characterization of the ethical obligations of physicians and patients, derived from the notion of informed consent, suggests an ideal version of the physician–patient relationship. However, this relationship seems to sit uneasily with a series of discussions about the changing moral landscape in the context of market reforms in the 1980s and 1990s. According to this set of discussions, the 1980s in China saw the end of political turmoil and the beginning of market reform, with the moral landscape shifting from collective to individual ethics, while the 1990s saw

[42] Cong, "Doctor, Family, Patient Relationship," p. 160.

[43] Nie, *Medical Ethics in China*, p. 144.

the moral landscape shifting from obligations to individual rights.[44] To the extent that there has been an expansion of thinking about rights and rights practices, this has unleashed a proliferation of obligations correlative to rights. However, as will be explained in the third chapter, a sociological consideration of the institutional conditions and requirements under which rights, i.e., the right to informed consent and the right to health in our discussions, are respected and protected will suggest that it is the performance of obligations, rather than simply rights, that better explains the operation of contemporary social and legal practices.

3.2 The Right to Health

The earlier section has discussed the historical trajectories of incorporating the doctrine of informed consent into the Chinese medicine and healthcare context. By using the informed consent as a typical example, it has sought to explain the differences between the Western (individualistic) perception and East (communitarian) perception of the right to informed consent and how the changing perception of obligation can help to address these differences. This section further explains two different views of the right to health, which seeks to explicitly explain that the two views of the right to health generate different types of correlative obligations to be performed by the state. The corresponding obligations constitute an "ecology of obligation".[45] As explained in this section, it is precisely the ecology of obligation that shapes and sustains the bond between physicians and patients as well as that between the state and citizens.

3.2.1 Ethical Notion of the Right to Health

Modern Western perception of rights, in particular a liberal view of rights basically views rights as equally possessed by individuals. As articulated

[44] Cheris Shun-Ching Chan, "Mistrust of Physicians in China, Society, Institution and Interaction as Root Causes," *Developing World Bioethics* 18(1), 2018, p. 19; *see* also Yunxiang Yan, "The Changing Moral Landscape," in Arthur Kleinman, Yunxiang Yan, Jing Jun et al., eds., *Deep China: The Moral Life of the Person*, Berkeley: University of California Press, 2011, pp. 36–77.

[45] Scott Veitch, *Obligations: New Trajectories in Law*, Abingdon, Oxon; New York, NY: Routledge, 2021, pp. 58–72.

by Fan Ruiping, "[t]hat one has a right to something means that one is entitled to it and ought to have it, independently of others' good will, permission, or benevolence".[46] As such, rights generate an obligation that must be imposed on others not to prevent the person from participating in the right. A liberal conception of rights typically sees a right as being equally and universally assigned to all individuals, without regard to the person's virtue, gender, race, class, and the like. The assertion of such a liberal right is premised on the notion that one is equally entitled to certain aspects of humanity, such as legitimate human needs, human dignity, and the like. However, the content of the liberal right is difficult to define and specify.

To illustrate this view, we can simply refer to the definition of the right to health as articulated in the major international human rights instruments. The right to health is recognized as a type of human right by the Universal Declaration of Human Rights (hereinafter "UDHR"), and it is reaffirmed and transformed into a right with legally binding obligations by the International Covenant on Economic, Social and Cultural Rights (hereinafter "ICESCR"). The content of the right to health can be defined by reference to an "overly broad interpretation of health", while it can also be interpreted by adopting a minimum core approach. The different approaches to interpreting the content of the right to health in different domestic contexts will be examined later, while a brief explanation of the vague understanding of its content in international law will suffice here.

Some international instruments take the expansive approach to interpretation. In the UDHR, the right to health is defined in Art 25. It specifies that "[e]veryone has the right to a standard of living adequate for the health and well-being of himself and of his family, including food, clothing, housing and medical care and necessary social services, and the right to security in the event of unemployment, sickness, disability, widowhood, old age or other lack of livelihood in circumstances beyond his control".[47] As also stated in the preamble to the Constitution of the World Health Organization (hereinafter "WHO"), "[h]ealth is a state of complete physical, mental and social well-being and not merely the

[46] Ruiping Fan, *Reconstructionist Confucianism: Rethinking Morality After the West*, Dordrecht; New York: Springer, 2010, p. 56.

[47] Art 25 of the Universal Declaration of Human Rights.

absence of disease or infirmity".[48] This understanding of health includes nearly all the aspects of well-being. It is pointed out by Norman Daniels that "[t]he WHO definition risks turning all of social philosophy and social policy into health care".[49] In this sense, this definition of the right to health is believed to be "so broad as to constitute an unreasonable standard for human rights, policy, and law".[50]

By contrast, other international instruments take the minimum core approach. For instance, it is important to note that there are attempts to identify the "minimum core obligations" which states should undertake to "ensure the satisfaction of, at the very least, minimum essential levels of each of the rights". The General Comment No. 3 introduces the "minimum core obligations" of the different aspects of social and economic rights. Paragraph 10 specifies that "a State party in which any significant number of individuals is deprived of essential foodstuffs, of essential primary health care, of basic shelter and housing, or of the most basic forms of education is, prima facie, failing to discharge its obligations under the Covenant". With respect to the right to health, the "minimum core obligations" are further specified by General Comment No. 14 in paragraph 43 as follows:

(a) To ensure the right to health facilities, goods, and services on a non-discriminatory basis, especially for vulnerable or marginalized groups;
(b) To ensure access to the minimum essential food which is nutritionally adequate and safe, to ensure freedom from hunger for everyone;
(c) To ensure access to basic shelter, housing and sanitation, and an adequate supply of safe and potable water;

[48] World Health Organization, Preamble to the Constitution of the World Health Organization.

[49] Norman Daniels, *Just Health Care*, Cambridge: Cambridge University Press, 1985, p. 37.

[50] Jennifer Ruger, "Toward a Theory of a Right to Health: Capability and Incompletely Theorized Agreements," *Yale Journal of Law & the Humanities* 18(2), 2006, p. 312; *see* also Lawrence Gostin, "The Human Right to Health: A Right to the 'Highest Attainable Standard of Health'," *The Hastings Center Report* 31(2), 2001, p. 29; and John Tobin, *The Right to Health in International Law*, Oxford; New York: Oxford University Press, 2012, p. 125.

(d) To provide essential drugs, as from time to time defined under the WHO Action Programme on Essential Drugs;
(e) To ensure equitable distribution of all health facilities, goods, and services;
(f) To adopt and implement a national public health strategy and plan of action, on the basis of epidemiological evidence, addressing the health concerns of the whole population; the strategy and plan of action shall be devised, and periodically reviewed, on the basis of a participatory and transparent process; they shall include methods, such as right to health indicators and benchmarks, by which progress can be closely monitored; the process by which the strategy and plan of action are devised, as well as their content, shall give particular attention to all vulnerable or marginalized groups.

However, even the above list of the "minimum core obligations" of the right to health is not uncontested. As pointed out by Tobin, "[s]tates never contemplated the notion of a minimum core when drafting the ICESCR... On the contrary, the realization of the right to health was expressly stated to be a progressive obligation". This means that from the liberal perspective, although the Western approaches to the right to health converge on the importance of health, it remains difficult to specify the different levels of obligations through the concept of the "minimum core obligations" correlative to the right to health.

The confusion view of rights, on the other hand, uses the language of virtue, emphasizing what I owe to others. In Confucianism, people involved in a close personal relationship do not see themselves as claiming rights and imposing obligations on others, while they may see themselves as engaging in a binding relationship of mutual obligations to each other. Moreover, as noted by Fan Ruiping, the key difference between the Confucian perception of rights and liberal perception of rights is that "Confucian virtue is inevitably intertwined with a vision of human flourishing, while a liberal right is an individual entitlement that is rightfully individual's irrelevant to any communitarian good".[51] The notion of Confucian rights suggests two points. On the one hand, a basic notion of Confucian rights can be used as "a fallback apparatus to protect legitimate self-interests when the virtues fail to obtain or people's personal relationships break down".[52] On the other, to the extent that the notion

[51] Fan, *Reconstructionist Confucianism*, p. 56.
[52] Ibid., 58.

of Confucian rights emphasizes virtues, it imposes obligations upon individuals to empress such virtues.[53] A Confucian conception of rights may impose different obligations on people with whom we have different relationships in different contexts. In other words, Confucian rights may emphasize specific, context-sensitive, and role-based rights. Confucianism can normally teach people to practice duties and virtues in common relations. The duties corresponding to Confucian rights are also derived from the roles assigned to them and the virtues produced by their intimate relations with others. From this point of view, Confucian virtues and their corresponding duties can be embedded in the pursuit of both self-interest and the common good.[54]

The Confucian notion of the right to health suggests that families should be the primary bearers of welfare and healthcare financing. Families must therefore support the financing of health care for their family members from their own savings. The principles of *ren-yi* are fundamental virtues. In Confucianism, humans possess the potential to pursue human flourishing in familial relations. In Analects, the quality of *ren* denotes the quality of loving others.[55] The human being who possesses the virtue of *ren* has an inner capacity of affection to love others, but to the extent that persons can hardly extend their love to everyone, they naturally express their love to their family members strongly while they only extend limited and weak love to strangers. The term *yi* denotes another important virtue. It has three meanings. First, in the Analects, *yi* means the ability to do what is appropriate. Second, in order to achieve what is appropriate, one should not violate moral commitments in order to gain material benefits. Third, the best way to practice *yi* is to honor virtuous people. In Confucianism, when the virtuous person is honored, his character can be learned and followed by others.[56] The combination of *ren* and *yi* denotes the following: "loving one's own family should be prioritized in practicing universal love, the pursuit of profit should be regulated by moral propriety, and the virtuous should be honored within social practices".[57]

[53] Ibid.

[54] Ibid., 60–61.

[55] Analects 12:22.

[56] Fan, *Reconstructionist Confucianism*, 76.

[57] Ibid., 77.

The obligations of the states are secondary in creating and sustaining a well-ordered healthcare market according to the principles of sincerity-fidelity (誠信). In Confucianism, Confucius uses the language of *cheng* by claiming that "if good men were to govern a country for a hundred years, they would be able to transform the violently bad and dispense with capital punishments".[58] *Cheng* is also emphasized as a moral virtue of self-completion in making himself/herself sincere without self-deception. In the *Analects*, the meaning of *xin* denotes that one must sincerely keep his/her own promises.[59] Furthermore, *xin* requires that one must dedicate oneself to the well-being of others with whom one is engaging.[60] When the Confucian notions of *cheng-xin* are taken together, it denotes that "moral sincerity should be promoted, the unity of words and acts should be maintained, and everyone and institution should be trustworthy in dealings with others".[61] The family-oriented market system does not support heavy taxation by the government; rather, it supports the efficient allocation of resources in the market. In order to maintain market efficiency and family responsibilities, the state functions as a market regulator, providing only short-term relief to the vulnerable groups who desperately need resources instead of long-term welfare programs. In this sense, the obligations of citizens, families, and the state generated by the Confucian view of the right to health are very different from the liberal conception of the right to health, although there is no universal understanding of this within the tradition of liberalism.

3.2.2 *Legal Notion of the Right to Health*

From the legal perspective, the right to health is a claim-right. Following Hohfeld's schema of rights, the meaning of claim-right which is used in the sense that "A has a *claim-right* that B should φ, if and only if B has *a duty* to A to φ", is well explained in distinction with the meaning of liberty, in the sense that the former has B's duty as its correlative, whereas the latter has the "absence or negation of the claim-right that B would

[58] Analect 12:11.

[59] Analects 1:5; 1:6; 1:7; 1:8; 1:13; 2:22.

[60] Analects 5:26, 12:7; Mencius 3A4: 8; Great Learning 3, 10; Mean 20:14, 20:17, 29:2, 31:3, 33:3.

[61] Fan, *Reconstructionist Confucianism*, p. 78.

otherwise have" as its correlative.[62] Saying that the right to health is a claim-right means that other parties are under obligations to support the right to health.

It is also important to note that the most important rights are claim-rights. This is well explained by Onora O'Neill: "most important rights are intrinsically relational in that they are *claim rights*, which mirror certain sorts of obligation: both claim rights and the corresponding obligations are a matter of required types of action, or of omission".[63] "The only exceptions are those unprotected rights sometimes spoken of as *mere liberties*".[64] For instance, to pick up a coin in the street is a right which is a mere liberty. In this case, no one has an obligation to let me exercise the right. In this sense, you (indeed all the persons who see the coin in the street) also have the liberty to pick up the coin. This is "different from my having a *claim right* to pick up the coin, which you have an obligation to respect – even if you find the coin first".[65] In contrast, a right of free association is a claim-right. This suggests that "[i]f anyone is to have a right of free association, then everyone must have an obligation not to obstruct free association".[66]

This is very commonplace to everyone. But it is not commonplace, when we try to distinguish between liberty rights and social rights. For some, especially libertarians, "universal claim rights *must* be liberty rights, and that universal rights to goods or services, and hence to welfare, are incoherent".[67] The reason for this is that "[g]oods and services have to be delivered at particular times and places, and hence by particular agents and agencies", and rights to goods and services can only be special rights which correspond to special duties.[68] In other words, social rights are not

[62] Emphasis in original. John Finnis, *Natural Law and Natural Rights*, Oxford; New York: Oxford University Press, 2011, pp. 199–200.

[63] Emphasis in original. Onora O'Neill, *Bounds of Justice*, Cambridge; New York: Cambridge University Press, 2000, p. 98.

[64] Emphasis in original. Ibid., footnote 2.

[65] Emphasis in original. Ibid.

[66] Ibid.

[67] Ibid., 102.

[68] Ibid.

universal or human rights at all. Rather, "[t]hey are only the institutionalized or positive rights of a specific social order or reflections of a specific contractual arrangement or social role".[69]

However, this explanation of the distinction between the structure of rights to goods and services and their corresponding duties and that of liberties rights and their corresponding duties is not accurate, because the distinction between the two only suggests that

> *if* there are universal rights to goods and services, then aspects of the corresponding obligations which have to do with delivery will have to take a different form.[70]

Further,

> [u]niversal rights to goods and services are quite coherent, provided that those aspects of the counterpart obligations which have to do with delivery are ***distributed*** or ***allocated*** to specific agents and agencies.[71]

The above two points suggest that the difference between liberty rights and social rights lies in their corresponding duties.

To understand the nature of the right to health as a type of social right, we must understand the idea of the "waves of duties". In general, Waldron's idea is that "the specification of the relevant rights is not supposed to be correlative to duties which already exist"; rather, it "is supposed to provide a *reason* for going out and looking for possible duty-bearers to undertake the tasks that these rights indicate".[72] In more detail, Waldron states that:

> We talk about rights when we think that some interest of an individual has sufficient moral importance to justify holding others to be under a duty to serve it. But if a given interest has that degree of importance, it is unlikely that it will justify the imposition of just one duty. Interests are complicated things. There are many ways in which a given interest can be served or

[69] Ibid.

[70] Emphasis in original. Ibid., 103.

[71] Emphasis in original. Ibid.

[72] Emphasis added. Jeremy Waldron, "Duty-Bearers for Positive Rights," *NYU School of Law, Public Law Research Paper No. 14-58*, October 15, 2014, p. 5.

> disserved, and we should not expect to find that only *one* of those ways is singled out and made the subject matter of a duty. . . . Even a particular duty, thought of as associated with a right, itself generates waves of duties that back it up and root it firmly in the complex, messy reality of political life.[73]

The above explains why there should be waves of duties correlative to a specific right. It is due to the moral importance of the interest protected by a right. If a given interest is of moral importance, it is unlikely that it only corresponds to one single form of correlative duty. It can generate different and various forms of correlative duties. Why is this so? Joseph Raz's idea of "dynamic aspect of rights" suggests that there are unpredictable and changing situations which may lead to new forms of duties.[74] Moreover, Waldron in the above reveals that there are many ways to fulfill a given right; and most importantly, there are many ways to support and back up the performance of a particular duty, which means that a particular duty correlative to a right generates "successive waves of duties".[75]

Let me illustrate this account by introducing an example given by Waldron. "The right not to be tortured... clearly generates a duty not to torture. But, in various circumstances, that simple duty is likely to be backed up by other duties: a duty to instruct people about the wrongness of torture; a duty to be vigilant about the danger of, and temptation to, torture; a duty to ameliorate situations in which torture might be thought likely to occur; and so on. Once it is discovered that people have been tortured, the right generates remedial duties such as the duty to rescue people from torture, the duty on government officials to find out who is doing and authorizing the torture, remove them from office, and bring them to justice, the duty to set up safeguards to prevent recurrence of the abuses, and so on. If these duties in turn are not carried out, then the right generates further duties of enforcement and enquiry with regard to *them*. And so on".[76] This example illustrates that the right not to be tortured generates a negative duty not to torture all persons,

[73] Emphasis in original. Jeremy Waldron, "Rights in Conflict," *Ethics* 99(3), 1989, p. 510.

[74] Joseph Raz, "On the Nature of Rights," *Mind* 93(370), 1984, p. 212.

[75] Waldron, "Rights in Conflict," p. 512.

[76] Emphasis in original. Ibid., 510.

but the particular form of negative duty also generates other duties to further support and back up the performance of the negative duty and ultimately to protect the interest recognized by the right. Further, the waves of duties must be allocated to specific agents. As O'Neill points out, "[f]irst-order obligations to respect liberty rights must be universal, but second-order obligations to ensure that everyone respects liberty rights must be allocated".[77] To better illustrate this, we may observe a list of the multiple roles played by states with respect to human rights suggested by Waldron:

(a) states are *parties* to international agreements and as *participants* in the global order,
(b) state power viewed as the *standard threat* to many rights,
(c) state power viewed as *a primary resource* for protecting rights, both coercively and fiscally,
(d) states as *guardians of national legal systems,*
(e) states as having *plenary authority* (background or foreground) over national economies,
(f) states as *coordinators of social duties and obligations.*[78]

The above explains the multiplicity of the tasks and responsibilities to be undertaken by states. The right not to be tortured generates successive waves of duties. In upholding this right, states are allocated to perform the roles involving the above (a) to (e).

The account of waves of duties illuminates that a morally important interest which is legally recognized as a right can generate waves of duties. When this account is applied to our discussion of the right to health which is a legal concept affirming the value of health, the right to health also generates waves of duties. But our discussion of the waves of duties correlative to the right to health is more complex than Waldron's discussion of the right to not to be tortured on two points.

First, in contrast to the waves of obligations undertaken by states ranging from (a) to (e), the right to health may generate waves of obligations ranging from (a) to (f). The reason for including (f) is that essential goods and services are needed to secure the right to health, the provision of which requires the state to "supervise the general system of

[77] O'Neill Onora, "The Dark Side of Human Rights," *International Affairs* 81(2), 2005, p. 428.

[78] Emphasis in original. Waldron, "Duty-Bearers for Positive Rights," p. 10.

(say) employment and pensions and health care, to ensure that private businesses in the economy play their part in this as well".[79]

Second, and more importantly, there are different aspects of the right to health. As noted above, the irreducibly communal aspects of the right to health should be distinguished from the individual aspects of the right to health. The reason for this is that, unlike the individual aspects of the right to health, the first-order duties correlative to the irreducibly communal aspects of the right to health must also be specified and assigned by institutions to specific agents of justice.

In sum, this section explains the content and scope of the right to health. It also attempts to clarify the interrelationship between the right to health and its obligations. The legal institutions for the realization of the right to health, as developed in the fourth chapter, will be the key ideas for understanding the relationship between doctors and patients, as well as that between the state and citizens.

[79] Ibid.

CHAPTER 4

Law and Obligations of Physicians and Patients

4.1 Informed Consent and the Obligation to Choose

What is missing in these discussions is an analysis of the link between marketization—medicine and health care as a commodity, taxation—and the right to informed consent. This matters as it is precisely this issue that reasserts itself in the context of healthcare reform, especially to help us understand the physician–patient relationship. Thus, in order to present a fuller analysis of obligations of physicians and patients underpinning their relationship, this section discusses the institutional conditions of health care—namely, the marketization of medicine and health care—played in changing the nature of the physician–patient relationship.

Since 1978, China had been undergoing dramatic market reform, de-collectivizing rural communes, privatizing formerly public enterprises and institutions, emphasizing individual responsibility, and permitting increases in social inequalities. To meet the overall objective of the market reform, a central directive was issued, which stated that "[e]conomic issue is the most important political issue; many social and political issues should be addressed from an economic perspective".[1] This objective was also applied in the health sector. The overall objective of the healthcare

[1] Huang, *Governing Health in Contemporary China*, p. 54.

L. Jia, *Obligation*, IPP Studies in the Frontiers of China's Public Policy,
https://doi.org/10.1007/978-981-99-6437-6_4

reform was to improve the supply side of healthcare services by developing well trained, highly skilled, and specialized medical professionals, emphasizing high-tech medicine, relying on curative and tertiary care, and focusing on urban health care, which allowed a great transformation of the healthcare system representing "the great reversal" of the physician–patient relationship during 1968–1978.

Specifically, a series of measures were adopted. In the urban areas, to meet the goal of "medical and healthcare modernization",[2] which required significant financial investment; however, fiscal decentralization made it impractical for the Ministry of Health to attain sufficient financial resources.[3] To address the financial difficulty, Document no. 62, as the first major healthcare reform document, was issued by the State Council in 1985, proclaiming the reinvigoration of public hospitals. During the period from 1979 to 2002, however, financial resources received by public hospitals were continuously reduced.[4] Despite this, the state still expected that quality health services could be provided by public hospitals in an affordable way. To meet the expectation, the Ministry of Health learned from the reform model of state-owned enterprises, with more autonomy given to public hospitals to improve economic efficiency. Public hospitals under the policy of "fixed contracting" were permitted to make profits from providing extra services after fulfilling their contracted tasks,[5] and they were also allowed to retain a 15–25% profit margin from drug selling to recoup the expenses of healthcare services.[6] Consequently, healthcare spending increased sharply with the average medical cost for an inpatient visit increasing 116-fold and the average expenditure

[2] Ibid.

[3] The Ministry of Health leaders expressed the "difficult financial situation" of both urban hospitals and commune health centers, the shortage of hospital beds and the lack of improvement in the living conditions of physicians and nurses.

[4] Before 1978, 50% of the expense of public hospitals was from the state budget, whereas the percentage reduced to 30% in 1980, 27% in 1985, 19% in 1987, and finally 6% in late 1990s. Shaoguang Wang & Peng Fan, *The Chinese Model of Consensus Decision-making: A Case Study of Healthcare Reform* [中國式共識型決策: "開門"與 "磨合"]. Beijing: China People's University Press, 2013, p. 63.

[5] In 1989 the Ministry of Health issued a document jointly with other four central ministries that reaffirmed the policy of "using the sideline occupation to subsidize the regular occupation", which encouraged the staff of public hospitals to set up industries.

[6] Huang, *Governing Health in Contemporary China*, p. 60.

per outpatient visit increasing 77-fold.[7] Government spending on health care increased at an annual rate of 14%, compared to the 18% annual increase for the total healthcare expenditures. The share of government healthcare spending rose modestly during 1979–1984, while after the promulgation of the Documents no. 62 it dropped significantly during 1985–2002.[8] Although healthcare expenditures increased sharply, the percentage of people uncovered by healthcare insurance was still high during the 1990s.[9] In urban areas, the percentage of people uninsured increased from 27.3 in 1993 to 44.1 in 1998 and continued increased to 44.8 in 2003.[10]

In the rural areas, while the CMS was written in the constitution in 1978, no effective remedial action was taken by the state to preserve the system. Due to the implementation of household farming and the reduction of state subsidies for the CMS, the number of collective-run health centers dropped from 390,309 in 1983 to 305,537 in 1985.[11] By the end of 1985, collective clinics were replaced by private clinics.[12] Measures were also taken by the state to tighten the regulation of barefoot doctors and private practitioners via upgrading their professional credentials. In the mid-1980s, the state started to reform healthcare insurance schemes. The new insurance schemes were financially supported by the insurance premiums that were assumed by individual households or collectives or both, and the insurance pool was also expanded to encompass towns. Different from the earlier compulsory CMS, the new health insurance schemes were voluntarily participated in. For CMS, however, the state allocated meager subsidies for it, dropping significantly from RMB 100 million in 1979 to 25.28 million in 1987, and the state even stopped funding it after 1987, consequently leading to the poor functioning of the CMS.[13]

What can marketization of health care reveal about obligations of physicians and patients to protect patients' right to informed consent?

[7] Ibid., 64.

[8] Ibid., 65–66.

[9] Ibid., 65.

[10] Ibid.

[11] Ibid., 54.

[12] Ibid.

[13] Ibid., 57.

First, to introduce the incentive mechanism of market into health care, the hope was that the market would provide healthcare services at reasonable prices and patients as consumers would choose good healthcare services at reasonable rates; however, the consequence was that when patients who were inherently vulnerable made by sickness and ignorance had to act as consumers in the medical market, their vulnerability deepened as they found themselves trapped in an economic mode of life which deprived them of actual options and information in the way that precluded them from prudent choice. Specifically, the obligation practices of the patient and the physicians were deviated from their ethical senses of obligation correlative to the right to informed consent. Due to the decline of free accessibility to medical and healthcare services, out-of-pocket payment at the point of health care was basically a common feature.[14] The transactions between physicians and patients were mediated by contracts. The contracts created some crucial legal obligations between the two parties—namely, the patients were required to pay, and those who were not covered by GIS and LIS had to pay by themselves, while physicians were required to provide medical services. This form of physician–patient relationship, and the bond underlying it, were thus created and sustained by "cash payment" or "no cash, no care".[15] The scope of information that was significant for patients was not restricted to the illness condition, the items for examination, the principle of treatment, medication the potential danger of different treatment, physicians' recommendations on the treatment plan, the items to be concerned about during and after hospitalization, the time for follow-up examinations, while it was also expanded to encompass the healthcare costs—including the names, prices, effects of the medicines and whether they were self-paid or covered by free medical schemes.[16] Even the patients whose medical and healthcare expenses were covered by labor protection services and those who received free medical service had to consider whether the health care and medicine

[14] Therese Hesketh &Wei Xing Zhu, "Health in China: The Healthcare Market," *BMJ* 314(7094), 1997, p. 1616.

[15] Indeed, there were once measures taken to improve accessibility for poor people to receive health care, such as phased payment and a green channel to allow seriously sick patients to receive treatment and pay later. These measures, however, did not work well because some patients avoided payment after receiving health care. As a result, almost all hospitals insisted on cash payment before the start of inpatient care.

[16] Cong, "Doctor-Family-Patient Relationship," p. 154.

were covered by the insurance, and physicians also needed to inform them of the scope of their free access to medicine and health care. Physicians were obliged to be informed not simply medical facts—the diagnosis and prognosis of patients, the nature of the proposed medical treatment, the risks and benefits of the medical treatment, and reasonable alternatives for the medical treatment—but also the cost of the proposed medical treatment. The performance of this set of obligation was out of the financial motivations of physicians and hospitals. When medical or healthcare bills were unpaid, it was often required by hospitals that attending physicians or departments concerned to cover the costs. This was especially so in hospitals and clinics in poor areas. Patients could rarely amass sufficient information on actual costs of treatments to make good decisions. The expansion of disclosure obligations was mainly to avoid potential conflict of interests, thereby reducing the possibility of being dissatisfied, complained, and even sued by patients as well as their family members. Physicians might discharge the obligations to inform and to communicate with patients as well as their family members, but they did not disclose all the information on the actual conditions and tended to exaggerate the seriousness of the patients' conditions. This was to ensure that when surgeries were not successful the patient's family members could accept bad outcomes, while when the surgeries were successful patients and their family members would appreciate and even show great gratitude to physicians. Thus, while the notion of informed consent was supposed to increase patient autonomy, in reality it did not expose patients to the accurate information about treatment costs.

How might the obligation practices of physicians described above fit within the marketization of health care and medicine? At a general level, the state's retreat from public provision of health care was supposed to increase the autonomy of public hospitals, but in reality it simultaneously produced the susceptibility of patients and their family members to market forces—over which not only patients and physicians but also public hospitals have no autonomous control. As noted, after 1978, rather than having a direct control over public hospitals, the state weakened its supervision for healthcare provision and increased the autonomy of public hospitals through introducing a contracted management system.[17] The contracted management system introduced the mechanisms of market economy to

[17] M Ramesh, Xun Wu & Alex Jingwei He, "Health Governance and Healthcare Reforms in China," *Health Policy and Planning* 29(6), 2014, p. 668.

health care, thereby public hospitals had to assume losses by themselves, and the amount of bonus received by physicians depended on the revenue of hospitals generated and bonuses were only given to medical professionals whose work reached or exceeded quantity standards.[18] The obligations to make discretion about how to allocate the resources to provide medicine and health care and the associated management were shifted to public hospitals, rather than the state—the sole obligation of which appeared to provide a limited amount of money to hospitals. Public hospitals therefore tended to increase their revenue by increasing the use of high-tech equipment, the provision of medical services, and the prescription of pharmaceuticals.[19] One major share of their revenue came from pharmaceutical costs, which accounted for 60%.[20] The mark-up of pharmaceutical prices by 15% were allowed for Western drugs and 25% for Chinese traditional drugs. Public hospitals were thus incentivized to prescribe expensive yet unnecessary medicines. As shown by study findings, "drug costs accounted for 60% of the hospital cost and generated a major share of hospital revenue".[21] This particular set of institutional conditions transformed our common understanding of what public hospitals are obliged to do. Public hospitals were obliged to maximize their profits, while physicians were obligated by thinking and acting as running some sort of small businessmen. As observed by a Chinese anthropologist, "the earlier image of the physician as a benevolent savior was replaced by an image of a profit-driven service provider who takes advantage of innocent and vulnerable patients".[22] Consequently, in the age of marketization corporate mentalities spread to public hospitals and physicians.

Sickness and ignorance made patients inherently vulnerable. When patients had to further act as consumers, their vulnerability deepened

[18] Xingzhu Liu & William C.L. Hsiao, "The Cost Escalation of Social Health Insurance Plans in China: Its Implication for Public Policy," *Social Science & Medicine* 41(8), 1982, p. 1100.

[19] Ibid.

[20] Ibid.

[21] Ibid.

[22] Yunxiang Yan, "The Ethics and Politics of Patient-Physician Mistrust in Contemporary China," *Developing World Bioethics* 18(1), 2017, p. 10; *see* also Cheris Shun-Ching Chan, "Mistrust of Physicians in China: Society, Institution, and Interaction as Root Causes," *Developing World Bioethics* 18(1), 2018.

as they found themselves trapped in an economic mode of life which deprived them of options and actual information which precluded them from prudent choice. Where there arose a new culture of consumerism in the sense that "all kinds of goods [were] available to whoever had the purchasing power", health care and medicine were also characterized as commodities which were not free of charge any more.[23] Although the notion of informed consent demanded patient to choose among a range of options, their choice was not autonomous in that it was highly constrained by their purchasing power. Some patients even had to seek healthcare services from unlicensed physicians and outside major hospitals at a reduced rate.[24]

Second, as suggested by the first point, the obligation practices of physicians and patients point to an understanding of the physician–patient relationship different from the ethical one as identified earlier. How did law and legal institutions in China respond to patients' vulnerabilities?

Before the promulgation of the 2009 Tort Liability Law, there were two ways of protecting the right to informed consent. The first was offered by three pieces of medical administrative regulation, i.e., the Regulation on Medical Institutions (1994),[25] the Law on Practicing Doctors (1998),[26] and the 2002 Regulation.[27] Two sets of legal mechanisms were established. On the one hand, the regime of administrative liability for medical disputes was established by the 1987 Rules on the Handling of Medical Accidents (醫療事故處理辦法). It was reformed by the 2002 Medical Accident Regulations (醫療事故處理條例). The two documents were administrative regulations issued by State Council. When the 1987 Rules on the Handling of Medical Accidents were issued, healthcare services were part of the welfare system in China and the majority of hospitals were state-owned. The 1987 Medical Accident Rules established a formal system of liability for medical accidents in which compensation claims were made against healthcare administration for

[23] "Introduction: Ramaking the Moral Person in a New China," in Arthur Kleinman, Yunxiang Yan, Jing Jun, et al. eds. *Deep China: The Moral Life of the Person*. Berkeley: University of California Press, 2011, p. 18.

[24] Liebman, "Malpractice Mobs," pp. 226–7.

[25] Art 33 of the Regulation on Medical Institutions.

[26] Art 26 of the Law on Practicing Doctors.

[27] Art 11 of the 2002 Regulation.

mediation or adjudication. Art 11 of the Rules on the Handling of Medical Accidents provided an option of hearing before a court when the two parties of medical disputes were not satisfied with the decisions made by administrative agencies, such as the Medical Accident Technical Appraisal Committee and the Health Administrative Department.[28] The Court may apply the 1987 Rules on the Handling of Medical Accidents instead of ordinary principles of civil law or tortuous liability to deal with medical disputes.

As explained by Zhu Wang and Ken Oliphant, the enactment of the 1987 Rules of Handling of Medical Accidents immediately after the General Provisions of Civil Law (GPCL) was to exclude the application of tortuous liability and limit the amount of compensations for harms caused by medical accidents.[29] Under the administrative liability system, a dispute about compensations for harms was a medical accident, referring to "a situation where the patient suffered death, disability, or organ damage resulting in dysfunction, as a direct result of fault in diagnosis, medical treatment, or nursing on the part of medical personnel".[30] Medical accidents include "Malpractice accidents", which refer to accidents caused by medical professionals as a result of violating administrative rules or procedures for diagnosis and treatment, and "technical accidents", which refer to accidents caused by medical professionals due to the negligence rather than violating any rules or procedures for diagnosis and treatment. Medical accident malpractice may give rise to administrative sanctions,

[28] Art 11 of the Rules on the Handling of Medical Accidents stipulates that patients and their families and medical units on the confirmation and treatment of medical accidents or incidents in dispute may be submitted to the local Medical Accident Technical Appraisal Committee for identification and settled by the health administrative departments. The decisions made by the Medical Accident Technical Appraisal Committee or the health administrative department is not satisfied with the treatment, the patient and his family and the medical unit may, within fifteen days from the date of receipt of the conclusions or treatment notice, apply for re-appraisal to the Medical Accident Technical Appraisal Committee or apply for reconsideration at the higher level of the health administrative department; they may also be directly appealed to the local people's courts.

[29] Zhu Wang and Ken Oliphant, "Yangge Dance: The Rhythm of Liability for Medical Malpractice in the People's Republic of China," *Chicago-Kent Law Review* 87(1), 2001, p. 29.

[30] Art 2 of the Rules on the Handling of Medical Accidents.

including dismal, warning or demotion to responsible medical professionals, whereas technical accidents only involve sanctions that are less severe.[31]

The second approach was provided by the General Principles of Civil Law (hereinafter "GPCL") implemented in 1987. Given that the compensations paid by the administrative liability were low, the Supreme People's Court (hereinafter "SPC") allowed patients and their family members to resort to compensations caused by medical professionals and bring their claims to court on the basis of tortuous liability under the GPCL.[32] According to the reply issued by the SPC to the Tianjin High Court in 1992, the SPC allowed local courts to properly deal with medical accidents in accordance with either the 1987 Rules on the Handling of Medical Accidents together with its implementation rules or the rules of the GPCL. The courts showed a preference to applying the GPCL since the reply was issued. In 2003, when the SPC issued another "Notice on the Trial of Civil Cases Involving Medical Disputes with Reference to the Medical Accident Regulations", establishing a dual system of administrative and civil liability to deal with medical malpractice.[33]

There are also two parallel systems of administrative and civil liabilities for violating the right to informed consent. The first set is a series of regulations of medical professionals, which provides for the obligations of physicians to inform and seek consent from patients. Art 26 of the Regulation on Medical Institution (執業醫師法) specifies the manner in which physicians ought to perform their obligations. It provides that physicians ought to explain to patients when surgery, special examination, or special treatment is taken, and they ought to avoid negative influences on patients. Art 33 of the Regulation on Medical Institution issued by State Council in 1994 (醫療機構管理條例) stipulates that the medical institutions should obtain the consent of patients and their family members or relatives when administering operations, special examination, or special

[31] ArtS 20 and 21 of the Rules on the Handing of Medical Accidents.

[32] "Reply from the Supreme People's Court on the Application of Law in the Case of Li Xinrong v. Tianjin Second Medical College Hospital for Medical Accident Compensation" [最高人民法院關於李新榮訴天津市第二醫學院附屬醫院醫療事故賠償一案如何適用法律問題的復函].

[33] Notice of the Supreme People's Court on Judging Civil Cases of Medical Disputes with Reference to the Regulation on Handling of Medical Accidents [最高人民法院關於參照《醫療事故處理條例》審理醫療糾紛民事案件的通知].

treatment. Art 11 of the Regulation on the Handling of Medical Accidents issued in 2002 by the State Council (醫療事故處理條例) provides that medical institutions and medical practitioners ought to truthfully inform patients of their conditions, treatment measures, medical risks, and other information when they provide medical treatment. Thus, the regulations in China have recognized the respect and protection of patients' right to be informed of their conditions, alternatives of medical plans and treatment, etc., so as to ensure that patients and their family members can effectively make their choice.

The second set of legal institutions to protect patients from vulnerabilities of their relatively unequal relations with physicians is the consumers' law. Art 16 of Rules of Implementing Consumer Law was issued by the People's Congress Standing Committee in Guandong Province. Art 25 and Art 26 of the Rules of Implementing Consumer Law was issued by the People's Congress Standing Committee in Zhejiang Province, Art 11 of the Rules of Implementing Consumer Law, etc. These articles recognize the protection of patient's right to health and the right to life by reference to the consumer law.

The problems with the regulations of medical professionals are that they do not devote any standard to detail the pivotal issue of how to establish the notion of informed consent. The vagueness of these regulations can be observed from the expression of the aforementioned provisions. One particular problem is that they do not specify the standards for determining the scope of information disclosure and the compensations for the violation. Their ambiguity can also be illustrated in the judicial practices of local courts, which was heard by the intermediate court of Zhuhai City (hereinafter "Court") in 2004.[34]

In this case, the Court found the physician and Zhuhai Hospital of Guangdong Provincial Hospital of Traditional Chinese Medicine had negligence in failing to perform the obligation to inform patients of necessary care after surgery. The Court also found causation between the negligence and personal injury caused to the patient. When dealing with the application of law, the Court held that 2003 Notice of the SPC stipulated that medical negligence should be dealt with by the GPCL, but

[34] Yan Longming and Others v Zhuhai Hospital of Guangdong Provincial Hospital of Traditional Chinese Medicine [嚴龍明等與廣東省中醫院珠海醫院非醫療事故損害賠償糾紛上訴案].

given that Art 119 of the GPCL did not devote any details to the standards of determining compensation, the compensation should be decided in accordance with the Consumer Law. In this case, the Court's application of the Consumer Law was to determine compensation so as to rectify the limitation of the GPCL in failing to specify the standards of determining compensations.

Two observations are worth noting. First, the administrative regulations dealing with medical disputes were in favor of hospitals. Before the promulgation of 2009 Tort Liability Law, medical disputes were governed by two systems, i.e., administrative liability and tort liability. The system of administrative liability was constituted by the 1987 Rules on the Handling of Medical Accidents and the 2002 Regulations on the Handling of Medical Accidents, while the system of tort liability referred to the rulings of the SPC in 2002–2003. As illustrated by the foregoing case, expert authentication (identification) played a highly influential, although not decisive, role in establishing causation. Expert authentication was governed by two tracks—namely, medical review boards dealing with administrative liability and judicial inspection agencies dealing with tort liability. Pursuant to the 1987 Rules, compensation could be obtained from the defendant who was held liable for medical accidents, which included both malpractice accidents and technical accidents and which was defined as "an error causing personal injury to a patient that results from medical personnel negligently violating relevant laws, administrative regulations, rules, standards governing medical care, or ordinary practice".[35] Under the Rules of 1987, the burden of proof was placed on patients, and the process of technical authentication was also biased toward hospitals.[36] Pursuant to the Rules 1987, when a medical accident occurred, a specific person should be assigned by the hospital to keep related original materials properly. In reality, however, it was very likely for hospitals to alter, conceal, or destroy the materials. It was thus difficult for patients to meet the burden of proof. The technical authentication organized by local health departments was also biased toward hospitals which were still owned by the state. The Rules of 2002, as a new regime of administrative regulations replacing the 1987 Rules, basically

[35] Art 2 of the Regulations, translation quoted from Liebman, "Malpractice Mobs," p. 193.

[36] Ibid., 194.

maintained the features of the 1987 Rules. For instance, the burden of proof was still put on the patient. Some improvements were made toward a better protection of patients. For instance, it was medical associations rather than health administrative departments that were responsible for organizing technical authentication. In spite of the improvements, the determinations made by medical associations, which entirely consisted of local doctors, were still believed to be biased toward local hospitals and physicians.

Both the 1987 Rules and the 2002 Rules, moreover, were subject to the criticism that the damages awards available under the regime of administrative liability were significantly lower than those given under the regime of tort liability. To seek a better compensation, many patients claimed for the compensation under the regime of tort liability. This was made possible by a formal reply issued by the SPC to the High Court of Tianjin in 1992, stating that "local court could properly handle medical accident cases in accordance with either the relevant provisions of the GPCL, or the State Council's Medical Accident Regulations (combined with the local rules implementing the Regulations), according to the specific conditions of the case".[37] The Notice on the Trial of Civil Cases Involving Medical Disputes was issued by the SPC in 2003, which explicitly established a dual liability system for medical malpractice. Accordingly, when the patient sued on the basis of medical accidents, the court would decide cases under the regime of administrative liability; while when the patient sued on the basis of medical fault the court would decide cases under the GPCl. Under the GPCL, the burden of proof was placed on the plaintiff; and, judicial authentication organized by the court was also introduced to rectify the problems of the technical authentication under the administrative liability regime. The reversal in the burden of proof and the introduction of the tort liability regime were more likely to lead to the decisions in favor of the patient.[38]

Second, the professional regulations and the judicial decisions demonstrated the ambiguity of Chinese legislations. The professional regulations adopted an encompassing term of information, while they left much room for judicial interpretation in discussing the issue of whether certain kind

[37] "Formal reply issued by the SPC to the High Court of Tianjin" [最高人民法院關於李新榮訴天津市第二醫學院附屬醫院醫療事故賠償一案如何適用法律問題的復函].

[38] Chao Xi & Yang Lixin, "Medical Liability Laws in China: The Tale of Two Regimes," *Tort Law Review* 19(2), 2011.

of information, for instance medical risks, fall within the duty of information disclosure. To rectify the ambiguity and inconsistency of the medical legislations, consumer law was used by local legislations to facilitate the healthcare providers' performance of the duties correlative to the right to health, including the duty of information disclosure.[39] Patients were perceived in the local legislations to be consumers to make choices on medical treatment, which was also recognized by courts. In the first case of artificial fertilization, the court found that the contract between the hospital and the patient was not explicit in specifying which medical treatment plan would be taken. The court held that given that the information regarding different medical treatment plans and their medical risks was essential for the patient to exercise choices, the physician's failure to explain to the patient about the change of the medical plan is a breach of the contract.[40] Although this set of judicial practices attempted to protect patients' right to informed consent via the consumer law, the obligation of information disclosure protected under the consumer law was consumer's choice rather than the choice jointly made by the physician and the patient. The key difference lies in the form and meaning of choice: consumer's choice denotes "preference amongst pre-arranged alternatives" which is "a limited form of choice with a limited mode of expression",[41] rather than the choice made by and through deliberative processes as pursed by the notion of informed consent. As mentioned, it is the notion of individual autonomy that underpins the right to informed consent; it involves patients and physicians with conveying and exchanging the related information, so as to make the decision in providing the best healthcare services to the patients, which thus reflects the ethical nature of the decisions. From this standpoint, the decision jointly made by physicians and patients are not meant to be equated with the obligations of the satisfaction of preferences, but demand discharging

[39] Art 16 of Rules of Implementing Consumer Law issued by the People's Congress Standing Committee in Guandong Province, Art 25 and Art 26 of the Rules of Implementing Consumer Law issued by the People's Congress Standing Committee in Zhejiang Province, Art 11 of the Rules of Implementing Consumer Law, etc., recognize the protection of patient's right to health and the right to life by reference to the consumer law.

[40] *See* the decisions made by Nanjing intermediate-level and lowest-level courts.

[41] John Tasioulas and Effy Vayena, "Just Global Health: Integrating Human Rights and Common Goods," in Thom Brooks, *The Oxford Handbook of Global Justice*, Oxford: Oxford University Press, 2020, p. 155.

the obligations of good communication between physicians and patients and decision-making for the best interests of patients. Thus while the adoption of the consumer law in legal practices intended to facilitate the discharge of physician obligation, it was in turn complicit in producing the commodification of health care and facilitating the decoupling of physicians' practices from their ethical senses of obligations.

4.2 Informed Consent and Tort Liability

This section identifies and discusses how the 2009 Tort Liability Law deals with the liability of violating the right to informed consent. The argument of this section is that although the legislative and judicial practices have attempted to adopt the patient-oriented standard to define the scope of information disclosure, they are ambivalent in making a balance between the patient-oriented and medical-practice standards in other respects.

2009 Tort Liability Law presents a new way of thinking about informed consent. It devotes two articles—Arts 55 and 56—to the notion of informed consent. Pursuant to Art 55, the obligations of information disclosure vary under different circumstances. Under general circumstances of medical diagnosis and treatment, physicians are obliged to disclose information regarding illness condition and treatment measures to patients; while under specific circumstances of surgery, special examination and special treatment, physicians have obligations to inform patients of medical risks, alternative medical treatment plans, and other information.

Art 56 provides for the medical measures of saving patients in case of emergency. Where the opinion of a patient or his relatives cannot be obtained in case of emergency, physicians are permitted, rather than obliged, to take medical measures immediately with approval of the person in charge of the medical institution or an authorized person in charge. Three points regarding the tort liability of violating the right to informed consent are worth noting.

First, the provision of Art 55 is ambiguous to the extent it does not specify the standard to define the scope of information disclosure or comprehensively list all the information significant to be disclosed to patients. While the stipulation is ambiguous, the scope of the information disclosure has been expanded by the Tort Liability Law. The obligation of information disclosure under the Tort Liability Law, as a law which has high legal authority, includes disclosure of alternative treatment options, which is not something embraced by all common law jurisdictions.[42] For instance, in the United Kingdom and Australia, while the obligation to disclose alternative treatment options is embraced by professional guidance, the legal obligation is restricted to disclosing medical risks.[43] As commented by a prominent medical law scholar, Zhao Xiju, "China is leading some other jurisdictions in the sense that it, through passing a piece of legislation that has high legal authority, has happily expanded the scope of information disclosure to encompass information of both medical risks and alternative treatment options".[44]

Second, to the extent that Art 55 is ambiguous, a narrow interpretation of Art 55 encompasses physician obligation to disclose a set of patient-oriented information. When Art 55 is narrowly read, the legal obligation to disclose alternative treatment options only applies to the circumstances where "surgery, special examination, or special treatment" is administered. "Surgery, special examination, or special treatment" refers to "invasive, risky, experimental, and expensive activities".[45] Physicians under the circumstance of proposing surgical or invasive treatment are obliged to inform of non-invasive, non-surgical, or less invasive treatment options. To propose risky treatments should be accompanied by informing of options with better risk–benefit balance or less risky options; experimental treatment should be accompanied by conventional treatment options; and, cheaper options must be mentioned when expensive treatment is to be performed.[46] What is noteworthy here is that medical costs fall within the scope of the information which is significant for the patient to make a medical choice. This category of information belongs to the scope of non-medical information that is considered significant from

[42] If Art 55 is narrowly interpreted the legal duty to disclose alternative treatment options applies to the circumstances where "surgery, special examination, or special treatment" is administered, which primarily cover "invasive, risky, experimental, and expensive activities". This suggests that physicians' recommendation of an invasive or surgical treatment should be accompanied with informing of non-invasive, non-surgical, or less invasive treatment options, risky treatments should be accompanied with informing of options with better risk–benefit balance or less risky options, experimental treatment should be with conventional treatment options, and cheaper options must be mentioned when expensive treatment is to be performed. Zhao, "Chinese Medical Negligence Law," pp. 440. 444.

[43] Ibid., 440.

[44] Ibid.

[45] Ibid., 444.

[46] Ibid.

a patient's perspective. To encompass this set of information suggests the Tort Liability Law's shift from a physician-oriented standard to a patient-oriented one.[47]

Third, while the enlargement of the scope of information disclosure suggests the shift to the patient-oriented standard, the ambiguity in specifying other aspects of the liability of violating the right to informed consent—for instance, causation and the burden of proof—implies the ambivalence of the Tort Liability Law in making a choice between the patient-oriented and the medical-practice standards. While the burden of proof and causation are crucial components to determine liability, the Tort Liability Law does not establish either the burden of proof or causation. A possible reason for the Tort Liability Law's silence on the assignment of the burden of proof is that it tries to restore the general principle of the burden of proof, which means that patients should bear the burden of proof.

If it is unclear about the assignment of the burden of proof in the Tort Liability Law in general, what is even more ambiguous is the assignment of the burden of proof in the informed consent law in particular. Despite the ambiguity of legislation, local courts have made clarifications on the assignment of the burden of proof in cases of the informed consent law. Beijing high court has recognized the distinctiveness of the cases of the informed consent law from ordinary cases of medical law, providing that the burden is placed on the hospital to prove that "they have explained to patients about illness conditions, medical treatments, medical risks, alternative treatment options, etc.". In this sense, while the Tort Liability Law is silent on the assignment of the burden of proof, judicial practices of the local courts have made attempts to alleviate patients' obligations to bear the burden. Despite this, the judicial practice of the establishment of causation manifests uncertainty in adopting the physician-oriented standard or/and the patient-oriented standard. Beijing high court has taken a physician-oriented standard, which allows experts (be they medical review boards or judicial boards) to assist in evaluating the causation between

[47] The physician-oriented standard holds that the physician's duty of information disclosure should be measured by the standard of a reasonable physician under the same or similar circumstances. The patient-oriented standard asserts that the physician's duty of information disclosure should be measured by the information need of the patient, so as to promote the patient's autonomy or the right of self-determination.

the act and the harm.[48] To establish the causation, however, it is far from enough to simply allow experts to assist in the evaluation. To establish the causation between the act and the harm, the court needs to consider this question—namely, when a patient had been informed of a particular medical risk whether he would have accepted or refused to accept the particular treatment. The consideration of this issue requires the court to further think about two categories of questions—how to establish decision causation and how to establish injury causation. The response to the former requires the court to decide when the patient had been informed of the medical risk whether he would have accepted or refused to accept the particular treatment, and, the response to the latter demands the court to decide when the patient had been informed of the medical risk whether the harm would be reduced. Experts are good at providing responses to the second category of issues by evaluating professional opinions, such as probability of medical risks, significance of medical risks, losses and benefits of alternative medical treatment options, necessity of medical intervention, and causes of harms, but experts are unable to assist in determining the significance of undisclosed information for a patient, the extent to which undisclosed information may affect a patient's decision, and the like. In this sense, when the court has simply recognized the need for experts to assist in the evaluation but leaves open about the scope of information disclosure that is significant from the perspective of a patient, its practice is incompatible with the ethical senses of physician obligation which would likely to support a broader scope of disclosure obligations. When a legislation of such a high authority is ambiguous, and the judicial practices related to the legislation are also uncertain, the problem with the legal protection of the right to informed consent is not only that the experts may be answerable to public hospitals and local health administrative departments, but there is no way to guarantee that the obligations are true to the patient's autonomy.

The foregoing discussion has demonstrated that attempts have been made by legislative and judicial practices to make tort liability available for patients to allege physicians' breach of the obligations correlative to the right to informed consent. Some of the judicial practices involving the notion of informed consent have explicitly adopted the patient-oriented standard, while others have been ambivalent in making a selection

[48] *See* Judicial Interpretations of Beijing High Court and Guangdong High Court.

between the patient-oriented and the physician-oriented standards. The ambivalence of the legislative and judicial practices may fail to meet the expectations of citizens. Such a failure may further aggravate the mistrust of citizens toward the medical consent law in China. As commented by Liebman after observing medical disputes between 2006 and 2008, "[m]edical disputes show how lack of trust in formal institutions—in healthcare, in the legal system, and in local authorities—is an important source of unrest. Medical disputes combine widespread distrust of the healthcare and legal systems with often severe harm".[49] He also argues that "medical disputes suggest that much of the institutional weakness, or flexibility in practice, is by design".[50]

In 2020, the Civil Code of the People's Republic of China (中華人民共和國民法典, hereinafter "Civil Code") was enacted. The Civil Code has devoted specific provisions for informed consent, specified the physician obligations and recognized the exposure of breach of informed consent to tort liability. Art 1219 of the Civil Code specifies the obligations of informed consent. The requirement of Art 1219 is different from that specified by Art 55 of the 2009 Tort Liability Law in the sense that the former requires an explicit consent to be made by patients or their families while the latter demands a written consent to be made by patients or their families. "Explicit consent" means that the patient or family member not only has to sign, but also has to clearly indicate their understanding of the treatment, which puts forward higher requirements. In previous medical practice, the informed consent forms were printed out, and the patient or the family member only needed to sign the signature without the necessity to fully understand the treatment. The obligations set out by the Civil Code require physicians to enable the patient or family member to understand the health condition, agree with the surgical plan, and actively request the surgery, etc., and ultimately sign the consent form to show that the patient or family member has clearly known and agreed to the treatment. In the foregoing analysis of the liability of violating the right to informed consent, from the perspective of citizens, as demanded by the corresponding ethical senses of obligation, the introduction of the doctrine of informed consent should be designed in a way that furthers the autonomy of patients in their medical

[49] Liebman, "Malpractice Mobs: Medical Dispute Resolution in China," p. 243.

[50] Ibid., 244.

decision-making. Further the autonomy of patients requires recognizing the goals and values of patients, and offering the patients the information significant for them to make coherent decisions according to their goals and values. The legal recognition and implementation of the doctrine of informed consent has further enhanced the expectations of citizens in expanding the autonomy of medical decision-making. However, when the medical consent law continues to be ambivalent about the adoption of the physician-oriented and the patient-oriented standards under specific circumstances, it is likely to deteriorate citizens' lack of trust toward the medical consent law, rather than enabling them to understand that some improvements have been made by the legislative and judicial practices.

4.3 The Right to Health in Courts

The right to health has been recognized by states in their own terms of constitutions and domestic laws in recent years. It has also received active support of key international human rights instruments, international organizations, and academic engagement all over the world. The right to health, as enumerated the ICESCR, correlates obligations of progressive realization whose primary obligations-bearers are the States.[51]

In realizing the right to health, States are obligated to fulfill both negative and positive forms of obligations. Some of the obligations are imposed on states to provide public investment in health services and health care. The World Health Organization has issued strong recommendations on the obligations of governments to increase funding for the provision of public health services. In the past, domestic taxes could be raised to respond to the needs of health and health care. Today, however, in an era of fiscal austerity, the capacity of governments to raise revenue is diminishing, while competition for scarce resources is intensifying. This is not unique to Europe. In China, similar questions are being raised: whether and to what extent public finance should support the satisfaction of the right to health, and how many resources should be invested in the provision of public health services?

Cases regarding the above questions are brought before courts in both developed and developing countries. Judges are called on to make decisions on the allocation of health service resources. In some developing

[51] Art 2 of the International Covenant on Economic, Social and Cultural Rights.

countries in Latin America, Africa, and Asia, judges have made decisions not only about access to healthcare, but also about rationing and prioritization of resources. When courts and judges are involved in resource allocation interventions, they have received a great deal of scholarly attention. The existing literature largely addresses the normative questions regarding whether the right to health is justiciable, in terms of whether it is subject to judicial review, and whether judges should be empowered to enforce the right to health.

There are three main reasons why the existing literature has focused on these questions. First, and most obviously, justiciable social rights can provide protection and enforceable remedies. Second, the justiciability of rights implies and even justifies a ranking of the importance of different rights. As noted by Jeff King, "the division of the rights into justiciable and non-justiciable sections can imply for some that the non-justiciable ones are subordinate".[52] An interpretation of *Viking* and *Laval* in the European Court of Justice suggests that the rank of social rights is lower than that of the right to free movement of services, in that the former is seen merely as a legitimate objective to be implemented by proportionate means, rather than as a right competing with the latter. Third, the justiciability of rights also strengthens the guiding role of constitutional commitments. This means that legislative and administrative bodies can be guided in their planning by the rights that are taken seriously by the courts. These three main reasons explain why much ink has been spilled on the normative functions of the justiciability of social rights, including the right to health.

While acknowledging the importance of the above questions, the focus of this section is different. Instead of analyzing the justiciability of the right to health and its impact on the enactment of related social policies, it examines whether and in what ways the right to health is being litigated in China, the United Kingdom (hereinafter "UK"), and India-including the cases of striking down related legislation and policies on resource allocation. Thus, this section offers a comparative study to discuss the function of judicial litigation of the right to health in China, UK, and India. It should also be mentioned that the institutional alternatives for realizing the right to health, including adjudication, are imperfect choices.

[52] King, Jeff, *Judging Social Rights*, Cambridge: Cambridge University Press, 2012, p. 53.

These alternative institutions are imperfect in the sense that the available institutional alternatives are not as perfect as ideal institutions might be characterized. But just as Ronald Coase says about economic analyses which compare an existing institution with an ideal one as "blackboard economics",[53] this section takes the real-life institutional alternatives, rather than the ideal ones, into account.

4.3.1 United Kingdom

The NHS in the UK was deemed by BBC as "one of the greatest achievements in history".[54] The reason for such a high recognition of NHS's achievement is that "[i]t was the first time anywhere in the world that completely free healthcare was made available on the basis of citizenship rather than the payment of fees or insurance premiums".[55] The NHS was established in 1946. Aneurin Bevan, the Labor Minister of Health, is generally credited with its creation. According to Bevan's reflections in the early 1950s, the NHS was created against the backdrop of the then existing market-based healthcare system and an intense struggle between socialism and commercialism. For Bevan, healthcare should be provided according to the "collective principle", which states that healthcare should not be seen as a commodity to be purchased on the market, but should be provided by health resources distributed free of charge according to the needs of patients.[56]

Against this backdrop, the NHS Act was enacted as a framework of legislation that sets out the basic scheme of the right to health protection. The courts in the UK interpret the right to health in a way that progressively channels and generates action by the state and civil society to protect it.[57] What is the specific role of adjudicative institutions in interpreting the right to health in the UK? To what extent can the courts intervene in the interpretation of the right? This section explains the

[53] Ronald Coase, *The Firm, the Market and the Law*, Chicago: University of Chicago Press, 1988.

[54] BBC News, "The NHS: 'One of the Greatest Achievements in History'," http://news.bbc.co.uk/2/hi/events/nhs_at_50/special_report/123511.stm.

[55] BBC News, "The History of the NHS in Charts," https://www.bbc.co.uk/news/health-44560590.

[56] Aneurin Bevan, *In Place of Fear*, Read Books Ltd., 2011, chapter 5.

[57] On the idea of "incremental protection", see King, *Judging Social Rights*.

role of the adjudicative institutions in interpreting the right to health in the UK. The purpose of doing so, as explained above, is to observe the interpretive authority over the definition of the right to health. To better understand this, it also locates the adjudicative institutions within a broader institutional setting and examines how other institutions may respond to the demands of adjudicating the right to health. The explanation of the institutional setting is necessarily sketchy, but it is sufficient for our purposes.

The NHS Act provides the basic framework that makes a welfare state possible. The laws are extremely complicated and have undergone a series of revisions throughout history, embodying the political compromises of democracy. There is a division of labor between the legislative and the executive branches. The British legislature has committees that help to scrutinize bills and the government. The committees are not just a group of civil servants, but rather an extension group of parliamentarians, which means that their exercise of scrutiny has democratic legitimacy, while it may also be subject to criticism aimed at democratic legitimacy. The administrative bodies, usually referred to as the government or executive in the UK, include departments (or ministries) and the civil service, executive agencies and public bodies, and local government bodies.[58] Local health authorities also play a very important role in the provision of community care. The division of labor between the legislative and the executive branches is also evident in the allocation of responsibilities related to the right to health.

The legal framework for health gives national and local authorities discretionary powers that allow, rather than compel, the distribution of public goods to protect the right to health. This differs from the legal frameworks in the areas of homelessness, social security, child protection, and the like, where rights and duties are explicitly specified. In this institutional structure, although the roles of legislative and executive branches, national and local authorities are created and limited by the health law, the demarcation of obligations allows for clarification. In the event of disputes, it is mainly the courts that settle them.

It was not until the 1980s that the first case on the allocation of resources to meet the right to health was heard in the UK. The first case was a challenge to NHS decisions on the allocation of healthcare

[58] *See* Paul Craig, *Administrative Law*, London: Sweet & Maxwell, 2021.

resources.[59] In this case, four people living in Staffordshire complained to the Court of Appeal that they were on a very long waiting list for orthopaedic surgery. The complaint was brought under section 3(1) of the NHS Act 1977, which provided that "[i]t is the Secretary of State's duty to provide throughout England and Wales to such extent as he considers necessary to meet all reasonable requirements (a) hospital accommodation… (c) medical [etc.] services…". Before the case was filed, the plan to expand the hospital where the four people were waiting for treatment had been delayed and almost abandoned due to limited financial resources. While the Court expressed sympathy with the complaints about waiting times for surgery, it ruled that the Secretary of State was not under an "absolute obligation" to meet all requirements for hospital treatment and equipment.

In subsequent cases in 1987 and 1988, the Court also held that it was not the appropriate forum for reviewing the allocation of healthcare resources, while the responsibility for reviewing and deciding such matters was delegated to public representatives. In the words of Christopher Newdick, this phase of judicial review in the 1980s was "passive" and "weak".[60] The passive attitude of judicial review was prevalent in challenges against government departments other than health care. This was thus an era "when the courts were more hesitant in encroaching on areas of policy making considered the proper domain of legislators accountable to the electorate".[61] This passive attitude of courts and weak judicial review were in contrast with the latter "active" and "hard look" phase during the 1990s.

In contrast to the passive attitude and weak period of judicial review in the 1980s, the mid-1990s witnessed a change in the attitude of the courts by providing procedural rather than substantive remedies. In Ex p A, D & G, the Court of Appeal (hereafter the "Court") clarified the procedural

[59] Secretary of State for Social Services, West Midlands Regional Health Authority and Birmingham Area Health Authority, ex parte Hincks [1980] 1 BMLR 93 (CA).

[60] *See* Christopher Newdick, *Who Should We Treat? Rights, Rationing and Resources*, Oxford: Oxford University Press, Chap 5, for a discussion on the comparison between "weak" and "hard look" judicial review.

[61] Christopher Newdick, "Promoting Access and Equity in Health: Assessing the National Health Service in England," in Colleen M. Flood & Aeyal M. Gross eds., *The Right to Health at the Public/Private Divide: A Global Comparative Study*, New York: Cambridge University Press, 2014, p. 118.

duties of the commissioners. In this case, A, D, and G suffered from transsexualism with male physical characteristics but female sexual identity. A and G were assessed as having "a clinical need for gender reassignment surgery" and D was awaiting this assessment. Under the National Health Service Act 1977, the regional health authority, in this case the North West Lancashire Health Authority (hereafter "the Authority") had "a duty to promote a comprehensive health service designed to ... improve the physical and mental health of the people of England and Wales".[62] However, this duty is qualified by reasonable assessment of the Authority, in the sense that "to such extent as [the Authority] considers necessary to meet all reasonable requirements", and appropriateness consideration in the sense that "[the Authority] considers are appropriate as part of the health service".[63] The considerations of reasonableness and appropriateness thus allowed the Board to exercise discretion in allocating its limited resources. In 1995, the Board developed a policy of deprioritizing the allocation of resources to those procedures that it considered to be of no beneficial health benefit. According to this policy, gender reassignment treatment was one of the lowest priority treatments. In 1998, this policy was revised by the authority, which included an appropriateness test for prioritizing treatments. This revision placed gender reassignment in the same category as cosmetic plastic surgery, hair transplants, tattoo removal, etc. The policy also explicitly excluded gender reassignment treatment from public funding. Although an exception to the blanket refusal was made in the case of "overriding clinical need" or "exceptional circumstances", no specific guidance was provided on how to determine such need or circumstances. While the three respondents expressed their distress, depression, and even epilepsy, their applications for public funding were rejected by the authority on the grounds of its limited financial resources. The Court found that the denial of the three respondents' applications was irrational for three reasons. First, the Court found that although transsexualism was accepted by the Authority as a disease during the proceedings, its policy still treated it as "an attitude or state of mind that does not warrant medical treatment". Second, in the sense that gender reassignment was not accepted by the Authority as an effective treatment for transsexualism, the Court held that the refusal

[62] *See* R v North West Lancashire Health Authority, ex parte A; D; G.

[63] Ibid.

to fund gender reassignment was "an indiscriminate prohibition of treatment". Third, the policy's belief that "gender reassignment treatment has no proven clinical benefit" was contrary to medical opinion that it was the only effective treatment. The appeal was therefore dismissed. The Court held that "the policy was irrational and quashed the decision not to fund the treatment".[64]

In this case, some general principles about how decisions about resource allocation should be made were clarified. First, the priorities for funding different treatments and the allocation of resources are a matter of judgment made by regional health commissioners within the statutory health framework that sets out their policy objectives and governs their discretionary powers. As noted by Newdick, it is inevitable the decisions must be made on discretion given that "[t]here is no all-embracing definition of what the 'promotion' of a 'comprehensive health service' requires".[65] Second, however, he further states that "the manner in which this discretion is exercised is subject to close judicial scrutiny".[66] This case also clarifies the principles of procedural fairness according to which discretionary decisions must be made. In establishing the priorities, the needs of patients must be compared in the way of "assessing the nature and seriousness of each type of illness", "determining the effectiveness of various forms of treatment for it" as well as "giv[ing] proper effect to that assessment and that determination in the formulation and individual application of its policy".[67]

These principles have been further developed in subsequent cases, and additional principles have been introduced to provide procedural safeguards for resource allocation decisions. In addition to the nature and severity of the disease, the effectiveness of the treatment for the disease, the South Central Ethical Framework further states that decision-making must also take into account the extent and likelihood that the treatment may work in each patient, the extent of improvement expected to be provided, the cost of the treatment, the number of patients who may benefit, and the relative cost compared to other treatments.[68]

[64] Ibid.

[65] Newdick, "Promoting Access and Equity in Health," p. 119.

[66] Ibid.

[67] R v North West Lancashire HA ex parte A [2000] 1 WLR 977.

[68] Newdick, "Promoting Access and Equity in Health," p. 119.

In addition, where the clinical evidence for a treatment is incomplete, the opinion of individual doctors must be given due weight, but it will also be weighed against other relevant factors. For example, in R v NW Lancashire HA, where medical opinion supports the treatment without reliable trials to support its effectiveness, the Court stated:

> [T]he mere fact that a body of medical opinion supports the procedure does not put the health authority under any legal obligation to provide the procedure. ... However, where such a body of opinion exists, it is ... not open to a national health authority simply to determine that the procedure has no proven clinical while giving no indication of why it considers that is so.[69]

In this case, the local health authority denied the patient's request for public funding, in part because of the lack of randomized controlled trials. However, the Court found that the balance of medical opinion, together with other relevant considerations, was not reasonable because large-scale trials could not reasonably be expected for transgender surgery, which does not involve large numbers of patients, and the medical opinion was not sufficiently considered by the local health authority.

Finally, in cases that decisions must be made involving weighting community interests with individual needs, procedures must respond to the needs of patients who have "exceptional clinical merits who will derive much more benefit from the treatment than other patients will".[70] These situations usually occur when "blanket bans" on certain forms of treatments must be weighed against individual needs. In practice, the UK courts "must acknowledge the differences in persuasive weight of, at one end of the spectrum, individual clinical opinion about a single patient and, at the other, the results of multi-center randomized controlled trials involving thousands of patients (and the gradations in between)".[71] This is for the purpose of guaranteeing that judges' sympathy with individual patients' needs do not undermine the general principle of fairness.

[69] R v North West Lancashire HA ex parte A [2000] 1 WLR 977.

[70] Newdick, "Promoting Access and Equity in Health," p. 120.

[71] Ibid., 121.

4.3.2 India

This section outlines the institutional structure that protects the right to health in the domestic context of India. It begins with a brief introduction to the Indian Constitution and then highlights the judicial activism of the Indian courts in public interest litigation (hereinafter "PIL") regarding the right to health.

Since the Indian Constitution came into force in 1950, the Supreme Court of India has been seen as an independent guardian of constitutional principles against violation and misuse by the government. The Court has also earned a reputation as an "engine of economic and social reform".[72] The Indian Constitution plays an important role in establishing social and economic rights as the goals of guiding principles for the central and state governments to develop their policies. The centrality of the Constitution in protecting socioeconomic rights, including the right to health, can be seen from the drafting process of the architects of the Indian Constitution in terms of recognizing the vast economic and social inequalities and the urgent need for corresponding institutional reforms.[73] Nevertheless, socioeconomic rights were not included as fundamental rights enforced by the courts. This was due to concerns about the limited judicial capacity of judges and the legitimacy of courts in terms of the separation of powers and division of labor to make complex social and economic policy decisions, rather than a negation of the importance of directive principles. This is because a wide range of social and economic programs have been implemented in accordance with the directive principles.

It was only after the end of the emergency in India that the role of the Court began to emerge and gradually became the hallmark of Indian jurisprudence. This role was developed by a handful of judges and lawyers through the model of public interest litigation.[74] In a number of cases, the Court has taken an expansive approach to giving meaning to the content of the right to life. The social determinants of the right to life

[72] Anashri Pilly, "Judicial Activism and the Indian Supreme Court," in Liora Lazarus, Christopher McCrudden and Nigel Bowles *Reasoning Rights: Comparative Judicial Engagement*, Oxford: Hart Publishing, 2014, p. 339.

[73] See De Villiers "Directive Principles of State Policy and Fundamental Rights: The Indian Experience," *South African Journal on Human Rights* 8(1), 1992.

[74] *See* Frank Munger, "Inquiry and Activism in Law and Society," *Law and Society Review* 35(1), 2001; *see* also Satyaranjan Purushottam Sathe, *Judicial Activism in India*, New Delhi: Oxford University Press, 2003.

were considered to specify the content of the right to life in the 1981 Francis Mullin case, in which the Court recognized that "namely, the bare necessities of life such as adequate nutrition, clothing and shelter and facilities for reading, writing and expressing oneself in diverse forms".[75] In other cases, the expansive interpretation approach was also used to give meaning to other fundamental rights in light of the principles of the Directive. This has also been the case with regard to the right to health. In *Paschim banga Khet Samity v. State of West Bengal*, the Court held that the right to adequate health facilities was also encompassed by the right to life. As the Court acknowledges, "[p]roviding adequate medical facilities of the people is an essential part of the obligations undertaken by the Government in a welfare State". It also further notes that "Article 21 [of the Constitution] imposes an obligation on the State to safeguard the right to life of every person".[76]

Resource allocation is therefore one of the key issues in the Indian healthcare system. This is a consequence of low public health spending, high treatment costs, and high out-of-pocket expenses. In addition, given the inadequacy of statutory obligations and the absence of binding constitutional obligations, courts have become important in structuring the obligations correlative to the right to be fulfilled by the state. To promote the realization of fundamental rights, PIL was originally conceived out of the need to facilitate people's access to justice and to initiate social change. It allows litigants to sue on behalf of a disadvantaged, marginalized, and vulnerable community, and as a kind of "speedy trial", it does not need to follow any procedural prerequisites.[77] The strategy of PIL has also been employed to promote the right to health. It was also clarified in this case that PIL is distinguished from an ordinary type of litigation where two parties raise and deny claims. As the court said in *P. Nalla Thampy v.*

[75] Mohini Jain v State of Kerala and Others (1992) 3 SCC 666 (India).

[76] Paschim banga Khet Samity v State of West Bengal (1996) Case No. 169 (Supreme Court of India).

[77] PIL was first introduced in Hussainara Khatoon & Ors vs Home Secretary, State of Bihar, 1979. The Justice Bhagwati, P. N. said "It is also the constitutional obligation of this Court, as the guardian of the fundamental rights of the people as a sentinel on the qui-vive, to enforce the fundamental right of the accused to speedy trail by issuing the necessary directions to the State which may include taking of positive action, such as augmenting and strengthening the investigative machinery, setting up new courts, building new court houses, appointment of additional judges and other measures calculated to ensure speedy trial".

Union of India, "The lis before us is not of the ordinary type where there are two contending parties, a claim is raised by one and denied by the other, issues are struck, evidence is led and the findings follow ...... The writ petition is essentially in the nature of public interest litigation and the petitioner has attempted to voice the grievances of the community".[78]

The jurisprudence of the right to health has been developed by the courts by invoking different rights. Certain aspects of the right to health can be chosen, such as the right to access affordable treatment and medicines and the right to reproductive health, while the rights related to the right to health can also be used, such as the right to non-discrimination, the right to employment of PLHIV, etc. In *Vincent Panikurlangara v. Union of India*, the petitioner moved the Court to seek "directions banning import, manufacture, sale and distribution of such drugs which have been banned in Western countries and recommended to be banned by the Drugs Consultative Committee under the Drugs and Cosmetics Act, 1940". This direction involved the withdrawal of 7,000 dose combinations of drugs and withdrawal of the manufacturers' licenses in producing 30 drugs. The Court recognized that the decisions involved not only technical questions about the harmful side effects of drugs, but also the interests of drug manufacturers, distributors, and patients. In light of this, the Court recognized the social complexity and technical nature of the decisions. Acknowledging that these issues could not be effectively addressed by the courts, it pointed out that it was the duty of the government to make decisions on whether to reduce the use of drugs with harmful side effects on the basis of technical advice from medical experts. While acknowledging the limits of the expertise required, the Court emphasized the importance of improving public health. As the Court said, "maintenance and improvement of public health have to rank high as these are indispensable to the very physical existence of the community and on the betterment of these depends the building of the society of which the Constitution makers envisaged. Attending to the public health ... therefore, is of high priority—perhaps the one at the top".[79] Thus, the Court called for the establishment of a centralized legal enforcement mechanism to strictly regulate the manufacture and sale of drugs and to eliminate harmful drugs from the market.

[78] P. Nalla Thampy v. Union of India, 1983 4 SCC 598.

[79] Ibid.

In this case, the Court also articulated the State's obligation under Art 47 of the Constitution to improve public health and the right to life. The Court said, it is "the State's obligation to enforce production of qualitative' drugs and elimination of the injuries ones from the market", and this obligation "must take within its seep an obligation to make useful drugs available at reasonable price so as to be within the common man's reach".[80] This statement emphasized that the State's obligations to maintain the availability and affordability of quality medicines correlate with the improvement of public health and the satisfaction of the right to life. In this sense, the Court in India has established the link between the improvement of public health and the satisfaction of the right to health and the right to life.

4.3.3 China

In the above two jurisdictions, the right to health is respected by the courts in the UK and India. In the two jurisdictions above, the courts intervene in resource allocation issues in different ways. In the UK, judicial review is used, as illustrated in the above cases, to extend equal protection to those who belong to a politically marginalized group. Courts have been asked to make a decision on how to represent the marginalized group. In India, the Supreme Court has also established the jurisprudence of the right to health by establishing the linkage between the realization of the right to health and other human rights and public health concerns. This section discusses whether control over the allocation of health resources has been given to the courts in China. In China, this section discusses whether control over the allocation of health resources has been given to the courts.

China signed the ICESCR in 1997 and ratified it in 2001. The Chinese government is thus required to fulfill the obligations set out in the ICESCR to progressively promote the right to the highest attainable standard of health by all appropriate means. In 2012, the Chinese government submitted its report on the implementation of the ICESCR in accordance with Arts 16 and 17 of the ICESCR. In the report, the Chinese government articulated its efforts to implement healthcare reforms since April 2009, with the overall goal of achieving universal basic health care

[80] Vincent Panikurlangara vs Union of India & Ors, 1987.

for all by 2020, covering both urban and rural areas.[81] Following the dialogue between the UN Committee and the Chinese government, UN experts from the Committee on Economic, Social and Cultural Rights (hereinafter "CESCR") issued a document expressing their concern about urban–rural disparities in access to social security and the social security of migrant workers.

The CESCR articulates its recommendations to the Chinese governments, including (1) to extend the coverage of social security, in particular to ethnic minorities, rural residents, and informal sector workers; (2) to take necessary measures to improve the level of social assistance; and (3) to follow up on General Comment No. 19 (2008) on the right to social security.[82] It also recognizes the general trend of increasing budgets for health services and efforts to improve health conditions in rural areas. It formulates recommendations for improving the right to health, including (1) taking all necessary measures to improve the health conditions of all residents, especially disadvantaged groups, ethnic minorities, and migrant workers; and (2) increasing the budgets allocated to the health sector and reducing the urban–rural disparities in access to health services.[83]

In the domestic legal system, the Chinese Constitution does not specify the right to health, although it provides for the obligations to be performed by the state in the Constitution. In China, the Constitution contains provisions regarding the protection of the right to health. For instance:

> Art 21 of the Constitution specifies: "[t]o protect the people's health, the state shall develop medical and health care, develop modern medicine and traditional Chinese medicine, encourage and support the running of various medical and health facilities by rural collective economic organizations, state enterprises, public institutions and neighborhood organizations, and promote public health activities".[84]

[81] Bertrand Ramcharan, "Implementation of the International Covenant on Economic, Social and Cultural Rights," *Netherlands International Law Review* 23(2), 1976.

[82] United Nations Committee on Economic, Social and Cultural Rights, "Concluding Observations on the Third Periodic Report of China, Including Hong Kong, China, and Macao, China," E/C.12/CHN/CO/3, 64 and 65.

[83] Ibid., 76 and 77.

[84] Art 21 of the Constitution of the P. R. China.

> Art 26 of the Constitution stipulates: "The state develops the disability prevention and rehabilitation undertaking, improves the disability prevention and rehabilitation system and its guarantee system, and takes measures to provide the disabled with basic rehabilitation services. People's governments at the county level and above shall prioritize rehabilitative services for children with disabilities, and combine rehabilitation with education".[85]

> Art 45(1) specifies that: "Citizens of the People's Republic of China have the right to get access to material assistance from the state and society in the event of oldness, sickness, and disability. The state develops social security system, social relief, and healthcare services that are necessary for citizens to enjoy these rights".[86]

In China, there is no single framework comparable to that of the UK. However, there is a very large number of administrative laws at both the central and provincial levels. The administrative laws at the central-level delegate authority to various administrative agencies in a dispersed manner. For example, China's most recent legislative enactments include the Basic Healthcare and Health Promotion Law of the People's Republic of China (中華人民共和國基本醫療衛生與健康促進法, hereinafter "the Basic Health Law"), which specifies the right to health and other rights related to health services.

In the four decades following the adoption of reform and opening-up in 1978, China has undergone a series of social changes largely based on market economy and economic growth at the expense of social rights. However, in recent decades, there have also been rounds of legal and institutional reforms related to social rights, especially medical and healthcare reforms. However, the role of courts in advancing the right to health is not emphasized. This differs from the medical and healthcare reforms in the UK and India. Comparisons between China's socioeconomic rights litigation, and in particular the right to health litigation, have been made by scholars.[87] As suggested by Randall Peerenboom, many positive experiences of Indian Courts should be learned by China,

[85] Art 26 of the Constitution of the P. R. China.

[86] Art 45(1) of the Constitution of the P. R. China.

[87] *See* Randall Peerenboom, "A Tale of Two Judiciaries: Judicial Enforcement of Economic and Social Rights in China and India," in Surya Deva, ed., *Socio-Economic Rights in Emerging Free Markets Comparative Insights from India and China*, Abingdon,

such as the introduction of "an increase in social justice" in terms of improving the conditions of the disadvantaged group, the increase of the "stature and legitimacy of the judiciary", "the provision of a safety value for disgruntled citizens to channel their anger in a peaceful way", etc. Some suggestions, whether learned from India or elsewhere, have long been taken into account by Chinese legal reformers and implemented in principle, while others have not been and should not be incorporated, especially in cases involving right to health litigation. Even though he notes cautions against the judiciary's active role in India, Peerenboom suggests (a) "an expansion of the jurisprudence of fundamental rights, and the creation of new rights, through the incorporation of directive principles", (b) "promotion of good governance and rule of law", (c) "the filing of the gap in the legislative framework and the stimulation of new legislation by the legislature", (d) "the facilitation of a dialogue between the judiciary and other state organs", (e) "the creation of another venue for democratic deliberation, arguably one less affected by the interest group bargaining that typically prevails in legislatures", (f) "an increase in India's global footprint and soft power as other jurisdictions, particularly in Asia, look to the jurisprudence of the Indian Supreme Court for guidance".[88]

However, the Chinese courts are different from the courts in the UK and India. The courts in the jurisdictions of the UK and India share a number of similarities in terms of their commitment to values such as the rule of law and the separation of powers, while they also demonstrate divergences in judicial reasoning in their practices. These similarities and divergences are precisely the reasons why China's judicial reasoning in right to health litigation is lacking. This is because the Chinese central and local governments have undertaken a number of legal and institutional reforms to advance the right to health. This suggests that Chinese governments are actively responding to social change and promoting the right to health. The engine of economic and social reform in relation to the right to health has essentially been the central government. However, the courts do not appear to have adopted a model of defending the right

Oxon: Routledge, 2016; Xiao Pan, "Realising the Right to Health: A Comparative Study of South Africa, the United States and China'," *Hong Kong Law Journal* 45, 2015.

[88] Peerenboom, "A Tale of Two Judiciaries," p. 131.

to health. In China, subordinate legislation must be reviewed in accordance with the higher law. If the superior law does not contain the right to health or the allocation of health resources, the inferior legal provisions are not allowed to create new rules specifying the requirements for realizing the right to health or the principles for allocating resources; otherwise, the provisions will be invalid if inconsistencies arise.

To explain this, we may simply refer to such an example. A farmer from Wulian County, Rizhao City, Liu Huanxi suffered from advanced lung cancer with brain metastasis. He was admitted to Zibo Wanjie Cancer Hospital for almost two months, during which 105,014.48 RMD was spent. After his death, Liu's wife, Xu Yunying applied for reimbursement for the medical expenses through the new rural cooperative medical system (新農合醫療系統) at the Wulian County Social Medical Insurance Office (五蓮縣社會醫療保險事務處). A written Reply was made by Wulian County Social Medical Insurance Co., Ltd. (五蓮縣社會醫療保險事業處) made to the application of the applicant Xu Yunying's cooperative medical reimbursement at Wulian County Social Medical Insurance Office ("《五蓮縣社會醫療保險事業處關於對申請人徐雲英合作醫療報銷申請的書面答覆》", hereinafter "the Reply"). The Reply decided it was not going to reimburse the expenses given that the medical institution visited by Liu Huanxi was not run by the government. Xu filed an application for administrative reconsideration (行政覆議) to preserve their rights. However, the government at the county level considered that the Reply was in compliance with related regulations. As a result, Xu filed a lawsuit with the court challenging the legality of the response and the relevant regulations under which the response was made. The court found that the second paragraph of Art 5 of the "Implementing Measures", which states that "participating farmers who go to the city for medical treatment must go to the government to hold a public medical institution", was invalid. It unlawfully restricted the rights of the Party in that it did not comply with the relevant provisions of higher-level laws, and therefore could not be used as a legal basis for administrative action. The court ruled that the response should be revoked. The court also ruled that other related regulations should be re-examined and dealt with by the Wulian County Social Medical Insurance Bureau. This case was a typical example of the right to health litigation in China, which demonstrates that legal provisions must be examined in accordance with the superior law, and the provisions are invalid when inconsistencies arise.

However, to the extent that the Basic Health Law promulgated in 2019 explicitly specifies the right to health, there is a framework law to realize the right to health in China. Art 5 of the Basic Health Law specifies that "Citizens enjoy the right to obtain basic medical and health services from the state and society in accordance with the law. The State establishes a basic medical and health care system, builds a sound medical and health care service system, and protects and realizes the rights of citizens to obtain basic medical and health care services". From this point of view, the Basic Health Law can lay the foundation for protecting the right to health in cases where the right to health is violated by administrative procedures. In other words, the Basic Health Law will leave more room for the adjudication of various claims for the protection of the right to health. Nevertheless, the engine for changing the law and policy on the right to health has not been the courts, but the Chinese central and local governments. In this sense, although the Basic Health Law has been made in China, the realization of the obligations as articulated by the right to health still require momentous modifications in the broader legal institutions in China.

CHAPTER 5

Obligation and Healthcare Reforms in China

5.1 Ethical Senses of Obligation Under the Basic Healthcare Reform

In late 2002, a mysterious infectious disease quietly struck Guangdong Province. This disease, known as Severe Acute Respiratory Syndrome (hereinafter "SARS"), later spread to other parts of China. The response to SARS exposed many weaknesses in China's healthcare system, such as severely limited public hospital manpower, funding, and facilities.[1] In 2009, the Chinese central government launched a new round of healthcare system reform, proclaiming the overall objective of this reform was that "every citizen is entitled to receive basic health care services".[2] On December 28, 2019, the Basic Health Law was promulgated. The overall goal of the health reform and the new legislation suggests three points regarding the topic discussed in this book. First, the Basic Health Law

[1] Shaoguang Wang, "China's Health System: From Crisis to Opportunity," *Yale-China Health Journal* 3, 2004.

[2] Opinions of the Central Committee of the Communist Party of China and the State Council on Deepening the Reform of the Medical and Health System [中共中央國務院關於深化醫藥衛生體制改革的意見] issued by the Central Committee of the Communist Party of China on March 17, 2009; Notice of the State Council on Issuing the Plan on Recent Priorities in Carrying out the Reform of Health Care System (2009–2011) [國務院關於印發醫藥衛生體制改革近期重點實施方案 (2009–2011年) 的通知] issued by the State Council on March 18, 2009.

L. Jia, *Obligation*, IPP Studies in the Frontiers of China's Public Policy,
https://doi.org/10.1007/978-981-99-6437-6_5

recognizes a number of patient rights and physician rights. The former include the right to healthcare, the right to informed consent, the right to privacy, and the like. The latter include the right to life, the right to safety, the right to dignity, other physician rights recognized by the rule of law, and the like. The Basic Health Law not only recognizes a series of patient rights, but demands a set of obligations to be performed by patients as well as citizens in general. Second, the Basic Health Law also stipulates that patients as citizens have obligations to promote their own health.

The third point suggested by the overall objective and the Basic Health Law is that health care and medicine are characterized as a public good to be provided by the state. As recognized by the Vice-Premier Li Keqiang, "the core concept behind healthcare reform was to provide a basic healthcare system as a public good".[3] The public provision of healthcare services was specified in the healthcare reform plan released by provincial governments. According to the reform objectives set out by some provincial governments, the universal healthcare insurance coverage was intended to be equal to and more than 90%, the objective set out by the central government. More than this, 95% of coverage of the healthcare insurance for urban employed and unemployed residents was proposed by other provincial governments, and 100% of that for rural residents was also proposed.[4] Moreover, the obligation to finance the provision of the public good should be assumed by the state. This has been recognized by the recently promulgated Law on the Promotion of Basic Medical and Health care, which promulgates that the state should assume the legal obligations

[3] Li Keqiang, "Continue to Deepen the Healthcare Reform, Promote the Establishment of the Medical and Health System that Suits the National Conditions and Benefits All the People" [不斷深化醫改 推動建立符合國情惠及全民的醫藥衛生體制] *Seeking Truth* 22, 2011.

[4] This obligation was intended to be assumed by provincial governments. The public provision of healthcare services was specified in the healthcare reform plan released by provincial governments. According to the reform objectives set out by some provincial governments, the universal healthcare insurance coverage was intended to be equal to and more than 90%, the objective set out by the central government. More than this, 95% of coverage of the healthcare insurance for urban employed and unemployed residents was proposed by other provincial governments, and 100% of that for rural residents was also proposed. Xin Gu, "New National Health Care Reform Enters Critical Stage," [全國新醫改進入關鍵階段] *Social Blue Book*, 2011.

to ensure citizens' access to basic healthcare services.[5] In this sense, the source of the legal obligations to provide health care and medicine for citizens is not the legal mechanism of contract any more, but a form of legal principle of communal responsibility—namely, that citizens should have universal access to basic healthcare services irrespective of means, while it is the legal obligations of the state to provide citizens a basic healthcare service accessible at the point of need.

5.2 Two Approaches to Healthcare Reform and Individual Obligation

As noted earlier, the healthcare reform plan and the Basic Health Law recognize not only patients' rights but a series of obligations to be discharged by the citizen and the state. This set of obligations concerns obligation's ethical dimension, i.e., what are the ethical obligations that citizens and the state should have. Bearing in mind the ethical dimension of the obligations, this section turns to two typical approaches to healthcare reform taken in China, analyzing whether, and to what extent, the obligation practices give true expression to the ethical obligations of the state and the citizen. Pro-government and pro-market approaches have been two major ways to reduce healthcare costs (especially over-prescription of drugs), thereby attempting to improve the quality of healthcare services.

5.2.1 Fujian's Healthcare Reform

By way of a typical example relating to the reform of public hospitals undertaken in Fujian province,[6] this section's purpose is to reflect on how this affects the obligation practices of physicians and the bonds between physicians and patients. To illustrate the pro-government approach to healthcare reform via the reform in Fujian province are for two reasons. First, it represented the situations of medical spending and socioeconomic development in China. Second, the implementation of top-down

[5] Art 5(1) recognizes that all citizens have an equal right to basic healthcare services. Art 5(2) further specifies the legal obligations of the state to ensure their access to the basic healthcare services.

[6] Before the national bailout of cost contain campaign, Fujian province was the single one taking administrative actions to reduce continuous cost escalation.

budgetary control over the operation of healthcare providers was also a typical tool deployed by the pro-government approach, which helps to reveal the problem with the pro-government approach in general.

The pro-government approach basically attempted to restore comprehensive command-and-control over healthcare providers and to carry out supply-side reform through providing sufficient financial support to public hospitals and cutting off the linkage between the income of physicians and market earnings. Thus, the reform of public hospitals was primarily to achieve cost containment and to change physicians' bonus system.

Specifically, traditional common-and-control mechanisms were implemented in Fujian province to reduce rampant cost inflation with a few supplementary policies functioning as monetary carrots and sticks. The decision for the reform was made by Fujian Provincial Health Bureau in 2004, with the issue of the document entitled "Fujian Provincial Health Bureau's Opinions on Further Containing Healthcare Cost in Medical Institutions" marking the beginning of the reform in 2005. Five control indicators were set by Fujian Provincial Health Bureau—namely, average expense per outpatient visit (hereinafter "AEOV"), average expense per inpatient stay (hereinafter "AEIS"), appropriate drug utilization, positive rates of high-tech diagnostic tests, and accuracy rate of service billing—to evaluate the performance of provincial public hospitals; while for the purpose of preventing local discretion or misinterpretation specific targets were clearly set with ceilings of AEOV and AEIS.[7] The province's mandate was penetrated through municipal health departments to public hospitals: municipal health departments extended the province's mandate to other first-tier public hospitals, the managers of public hospitals further allocated the quotas for cost containment down to different clinical departments, and within public hospitals the five control indicators were incorporated into their Hospital Management Assessment System (hereinafter "HMAS"),[8] which suggests that those externally mandated cost-containment goals were incorporated into the hospitals'

[7] Alex Jingwei He & Jiwei Qian, "Hospitals' Responses to Administrative Cost-Containment Policy in Urban China: The Case of Fujian Province," *China Quarterly* 216, 2013, p. 951.

[8] Although the structure and contents of HMAS vary across localities, a typical HMAS includes personnel, physical and technological capacities, efficiency, workload, as well as service quality.

internal assessment ones.[9] In addition to close monitoring, sophisticated overall evaluation was conducted by provincial health bureau and municipal health departments—with a quantified system evaluating drug procurement, prescription of antibiotics, workload, etc. The evaluation results affected the ranking and reputation of public hospitals; as a hard constraint imposed on public hospitals the revenues earned by public hospitals beyond the ceilings would be confiscated by health authorities and reallocated to other causes, such as medical education, rural health care, etc.; and, since 2007 the cost-containment performance was linked to the subsidies received by public hospitals.[10]

Public hospitals and physicians also assigned with revenue targets by the income system, which primarily came from four sources, i.e., drug income, treatment procedures, diagnostic tests, and government subsidies. In order to make profits, the income was monitored in a dynamic way by hospital managers, and benchmarked with the control targets of cost reduction.[11] Hospital managers under the dual systems manipulated the mix of drug and diagnosis and treatment to meet the objectives. To meet the target of cost reduction, high-tech diagnostic tests were cut off, while the revenue earned from drug selling was tolerated to ensure that physicians could still earn commission from pharmaceutical companies. Where there was a decoupling policy of income of drug selling from hospital revenue for the purpose of curtailing over-prescription, public hospitals under this circumstance were also likely to increase the volume of services to increase revenue.[12] In effect, physicians working under the rigorous monitoring and evaluation system were thus very likely to work under extremely heavy pressures.

The health policies aimed to achieve cost reduction, which required public hospitals and physicians to change their practices. The change of the obligation practices of public hospitals and physicians suggests a further decoupling from their ethical senses of physician obligation.

[9] JingWei He, "Combating Healthcare Cost Inflation with Concerted Administrative Actions in a Chinese Province," *Public Administration and Development* 31(3), 2011, pp. 218–9.

[10] Ibid., 219.

[11] He & Qian, "Hospitals' Responses to Administrative Cost-Containment Policy in Urban China," pp. 957–958.

[12] Ibid., 965.

Two points are noteworthy. First, contrary to the once settled understanding that administrative measures were unable to infiltrate the public hospital system because the health bureaucracy is insufficiently competent and the earlier administrative control mechanism had basically collapsed during the period of healthcare marketization, the health administrative measures were able to penetrate the public hospital system.[13] In the above case, while having to abide by the administrative mandate of cost control imposed by the health administration, public hospitals still engaged in various unintended opportunistic practices to defend their economic interests.[14] Physicians who were managed under the public hospital system were also required to change into corporate mentalities. A physician described the experience when over-prescription of drugs was prohibited by the government, whist public hospitals still tried to maintain revenue:

> The hospital demands that prescriptions drugs should continue less than 30% of a patient's total medical costs. This means if the bill amounts to 100 *yuan*, the cost of drugs should be less than 30 *yuan*. If it exceeds 30 *yuan*—like 45 *yuan*—the hospital will deduct the extra sum from my own wages. But, to get around the policy, one can order more high-tech diagnostic tests to increase the total medical costs. So a good doctor should also be a good accountant, always calculating costs.[15]

The increasingly demanding regulatory mechanisms brought by the public hospital reform and accompanying obligations incumbent on physicians did not dispel their economic incentives to raise revenues. The mentality of thinking and acting in the way that "a good doctor

[13] Huang, *Governing Health in Contemporary China*, pp. 81–2; *see* also William Hisao, "The Chinese Health Care System: Lessons for Other Nations," *Social Science & Medicine* 41, 1995.

[14] He, Alex Jingwei & Jiwei Qian, "Hospitals' Responses to Administrative Cost-Containment Policy in Urban China: The Case of Fujian Province," *China Quarterly* 216, 2013, p. 946.

[15] Jing-Bao Nie, Yu Cheng, Xiang Zou, et al., "The Vicious Circle of Patient-Physician Mistrust in China: Health Professionals' Perspectives, Institutional Conflict of Interest, and Building Trust Through Medical Professionalism," *Developing World Bioethics* 18(1), 2018, p. 33.

should also be a good accountant" distorted their practices of professional obligations in the way that prioritized maximization of economic interests.

Second, the regulatory mechanisms distanced and disrupted the bonds of trust between physicians and patients. The heavy pressure, overload, and limited time prevented physicians from performing the obligations to provide good communication with their patients.[16] The poor communication was the primary factor to ignite violent conflicts between physicians and patients.[17] The number of violent conflict incidents between medical staff and patients increased sharply from 10,248 in 2006 and only started to decrease from 2014. Physicians and patients were trapped in a vicious circle of mistrust. There was not only deep mistrust felt by patients toward physicians, but also widespread fear of complaints, disputes, and lawsuits felt by physicians toward patients and their family members. Physicians' mistrust of patients might lead to practices of self-protection. The use of unnecessary high-tech diagnostic tests and less communication with patients, for instance, were assumed as ways to avoid making mistakes and being involved in lawsuits. The physician practices of excessive use of diagnostic tests together with their ineffective communication exacerbated the difficulties in communication, which further gave rise to the poor healthcare outcomes. There arose, then, increasing discontent felt by patients. When the discontent of patients with treatment was reported by mass media in a negative, sensational, and sometimes irresponsible way, there arose strong feeling among physicians that they were not treated fairly and their work was not properly appreciated. Consequently, their strong sense of injustice, anger, and the mentality of victimization ultimately generated higher level of mistrust.[18] Thus, given that the institutional arrangements within the public hospital still distorted physician professional obligations in the way that prioritized the economic interests ahead of patient health needs, the rigorous monitoring and evaluation system and the accompanying obligations incumbent on physicians by the pro-government public

[16] He & Qian, "Explaining Medical Disputes in Chinese Public Hospitals; He & Qian, "Hospitals' Responses to Administrative Cost-Containment Policy in Urban China," 2013.

[17] *See* He & Qian, "Explaining Medical Disputes in Chinese Public Hospitals."

[18] For empirical research on physicians' view regarding the mistrust and distrust between physicians and patients, see "The vicious circle of patient-physician mistrust in China: Health professionals' perspectives, institutional conflict of interest, and building trust through medical professionalism".

hospital reform was not likely to discontinue the deterioration of the physician–patient relationship and to improve the bond of trust between them.

5.2.2 *Sanming's Healthcare Reform*

The second example is the health insurance reform in Sanming, Fujian Province. In the context of China's healthcare reform, Sanming's health insurance reform has been regarded as a model. Before the reform, Sanming's health insurance system was fragmented, with three systems covering different groups of citizens and providing different service packages. To address the lack of coordination and bureaucratic conflicts between the social security and health departments, a new commission called the Health Insurance Management Commission (醫療保險管理中心) was established to take over the management of three healthcare insurance schemes. Its establishment was aimed at overcoming the severe bureaucratic fragmentation and intense inter-bureaucratic conflicts that had existed for a long time.[19]

First, the consolidation of the three schemes increased the protection of insurance against financial risks. Second, to merge the 26 insurance management offices into one reduced administrative costs. Third, given that hospitals had to confront with a single health insurer with strong negotiation power, behaviors such as cost escalation were curbed.[20] In particular, two agreements were signed between the health insurance commission and public hospitals, whose content was regarding the content of the health services and ceilings for costs. The agreements held hospital directors to be accountable for the performance of hospitals, and also introduced a new measurement system to rate the performance of

[19] Although the healthcare bureaucracy is supposed to manage policy making and control agenda setting in the area of health care, severe bureaucratic fragmentation existed in the structure of healthcare governance in practice. Horizontal fragmentation involved different healthcare bureaucracies, including the social security bureaucracy, the finance bureaucracy, the personnel bureaucracy, the planning bureaucracy, the civil affairs bureaucracy, etc. Vertical administrative decentralization also created a fragmented healthcare system with hospitals owed by different levels of governments. Alex Jingwei He, "Manoeuvring within a Fragmented Bureaucracy: Policy Entrepreneurship in China's Local Healthcare Reform," *The China Quarterly* 236, 2018, pp. 1088–1110.

[20] Ibid., 1099.

hospital directors based on four categories of indicators, including clinical quality, facility development, operation safety, and cost control.[21] Physicians' income was decoupled from the profits they generated, and physicians' salaries consisted of a base salary plus a bonus based on performance, i.e., seniority, quality of medical services, quantity of services, and achievement of goals such as cost control.[22] What can the health insurance reform tell us about the changing nature of the state–citizen relationship discussed in this book?

One way to understand this is to understand Sanming's health insurance reform as an illustration of the idea of the public contract. Unlike a private contract between two private parties, a public contract is used as a regulatory tool to achieve certain specified goals. In the context of health care, a public contract can be exemplified by multiple long-term contracts between a variety of healthcare providers and third-party payers (social health insurers).[23] The Sanming reform adopted such a public contract. The public contract, which consisted of two agreements, was signed by public hospitals and social health insurance funds. The goals of the two agreements were to control costs and improve the quality of healthcare services. Sanming's public contract model separated the roles and functions of health insurers and purchasers, forming a multiple triangular relationship instead of the traditional single triangular relationship among insurers (purchasers), providers, and enrollees (patients).

The public contract was consisted of five relationships: (a) regulator—payer; (b) payer/health insurance agency—fund collector; (c) fund collector—patients; (d) patient—healthcare provider; (e) healthcare provider—regulator.[24] Compared to the previous single triangular relationship between insurers (purchasers), providers, and enrollees (citizens), this multiple triangular relationship involved a certain degree of decentralization and devolution. The payer–provider relationship was relatively independent of the direct control of government agencies, and therefore

[21] Hongqiao Fu, Ling Li, Mingqiang Li, et al., "An Evaluation of Systemic Reforms of Public Hospitals: The Sanming Model in China," *Health Policy and Planning* 32(8), 2017, p. 1137.

[22] Ibid.

[23] Edward Gu & Imogen Page-Jarrett, "The Top-Level Design of Social Health Insurance Reforms in China: Towards Universal Coverage, Improved Benefit Design, and Smart Payment Methods," *Journal of Chinese Governance* 3(3), 2018, p. 342.

[24] Ibid., 344.

the health insurance agency, as the payer, was able to exercise a number of contractual powers by monitoring and evaluating the performance of public hospitals (healthcare providers) in meeting the obligations set forth in the contract terms and standards. The standards and parameters were set to evaluate the performance of the directors of public hospitals, and the performance of the directors was directly linked to the sum of the salaries of all the doctors of the same public hospital.[25] The two levels of payment—the external agreement between the health insurance agency and public hospitals and the internal agreement between public hospitals and physicians—were linked in Sanming, through which the public contract was a regulatory instrument that combined central control through hierarchical setting of goals and parameters and lower-level coordination through devolution of management to public hospitals and physicians. Thus, the public contract was a centralized decentralization mechanism that combined with, rather than replaced, bureaucracy and hierarchy.

Second, it requires a rethinking of the nature of the physician–patient and state–citizen relationships as they have been transformed by the marketization of health care. In theory, the introduction of the public contract between health insurers and healthcare providers is an attempt to increase the role of insurers in the procurement of healthcare services from public hospitals.[26] Citizens are encouraged to participate in collective decision-making processes in which their feedback on treatment experiences and their choices about what kind of health services they want to receive are respected, as their choices and demands are collected and transmitted through health insurance companies to healthcare providers. However, as mentioned above in the case of Sanming, although some bureaucratic control is imposed on public hospitals by setting the standards and parameters within which public hospitals can compete with each other, citizens (both as patients and as enrollees who contribute to the operation of health insurance schemes) were still excluded from

[25] Jifu Zhan, *Comprehensive Reform of Public Hospitals in Sanming City* [三明市公立醫院綜合改革] Fuzhou: Fujian People's Press, 2014, pp. 16–17.

[26] *See* Edward Gu & Imogen Page-Jarrett, "The Top-Level Design of Social Health Insurance Reforms in China: Towards Universal Coverage, Improved Benefit Design, and Smart Payment Methods," *Journal of Chinese Governance* 3(3), 2018, p. 332; *see* also Winnie Yip & William C. Hsiao, "The Chinese Health System at a Crossroads," *Health Affairs* 27(2), 2008.

the regulatory processes, especially in setting the objectives of public hospitals.

Moreover, given this reality, the ethical sense of obligation for citizens to be responsible for their own health may only make them feel that they are simply self-sufficient individuals. Given that civic duties are based on the common need and the common good through mutual participation and mutual benefit of the healthcare system, the state's failure to meet the common need and the common good may make citizens feel that they are simply saving financial resources for the state. Since recent legislation has recognized the obligations of citizens to reduce their demands on the limited financial resources of the state, citizens are obliged to accept the consequences of their consumption of financial resources in the context of health care. If this is the case, citizens may also have high expectations that they will be able to make autonomous choices through participation in decision-making processes to decide how financial resources will be used, while in reality the state's performance does not meet citizens' expectations. Thus, there is a gap between citizens' high expectations of what should happen and the state's lower performance in reality. In this situation, the bond of trust can break down if there is no communication between the citizen and the state to clarify the misunderstanding. Thus, as identified and discussed in this section, while the systemic healthcare reform has sought to achieve the objective of expanding the bond of trust between physician and patient to encompass the relations between healthcare insurance schemes and citizens via the universal coverage of basic healthcare, the healthcare insurance schemes have been still incompetent and insufficient to perform the obligations and functions to realize the objective.

CHAPTER 6

Public Health Emergency Management and People's Trust

In China, although the right to health is largely a state obligation, the central government directs health policy and supports preventive health measures, leaving a high degree of flexibility to the health sector and provincial governments. The Covid-19 outbreak has posed significant challenges to the capacity of the state, including the rule of law, to respond to the pandemic and the widespread deaths, illnesses, and economic devastation. Unlike ordinary medical activities, public health management is inherently related to the state's capacity building. Public health is distinguished from healthcare in several respects:

> Public health focuses on: (1) the health and safety of populations rather than the health of individual patients; (2) prevention of injury and disease rather than treatment and care; (3) relationships between the government and the community rather than the physician and patient; and (4) population-based services grounded on the scientific methodologies of public health (e.g., biostatistics and epidemiology) rather than personal medical services.[1]

The outbreak of the pandemic requires the exercise of centralized executive power, but when executive power goes too far, it can be used to

[1] Lawrence O. Gostin, "Public Health Law: A Renaissance," *The Journal of Law, Medicine & Ethics* 30(2), 2002, p. 136.

L. Jia, *Obligation*, IPP Studies in the Frontiers of China's Public Policy,
https://doi.org/10.1007/978-981-99-6437-6_6

trample on liberty. Accordingly, public health law involves the legal duties and powers of the executive to pursue the highest possible level of public health and to limit the exercise of its power to protect privacy, liberty, and other legally protected rights of individuals.[2]

In response to infectious diseases, outbreak management relies on liberal and autocratic measures. Both liberal democracies and autocratic regimes may use a combination of these measures. In some autocratic regimes, such as Singapore and Vietnam, their relative effectiveness in containing the spread of Covid-19 appears to have depended on non-autocratic elements of public health emergency management—carefully restricted measures in Singapore and open and transparent management in Vietnam.[3]

This situation has been captured by Francis Fukuyama, observing that "[s]ome democracies have performed well, but others have not, and the same is true for autocracies", and thus not "a matter of regime type".[4] The rule of law is not a binary condition; rather, "legal systems are medium- to low-specificity activities with high transaction volumes".[5] The rule of law is not just law and legal institutions, but also involves the mechanisms across the entire state. The factors responsible for successful public health emergency management are many; state capacity is a major one. The state capacity has been discussed in recent literature regarding the Chinese government at a general level and the Chinese government's responses to the Covid-19 outbreak.[6] These discussions have

[2] Ibid.

[3] *See* Trang (Mae) Nguyen, "Vietnam's Astonishing Success at Curbing Covid-19 Outbreaks," *The Regulatory Review—Opinion*, 2020.

[4] Fukuyama Francis, "The Pandemic and Political Order," *Foreign Affairs* 99, 2020, https://www.foreignaffairs.com/articles/world/2020-06-09/pandemic-and-political-order.

[5] On the one hand, while state power refers to the state's capacities to mobilize resources, the rule of law relates to "governance through law", rather than through decree or management—the rule of law is largely dependent on the resource mobilization of the state. On the other hand, the rule of law "is an ideal designed to correct dangers of abuse that arise in general when political power is exercised, not dangers of abuse that arise from law in particular", the rule of law also exercises restraints on the exercise of the state power. Jeremy Waldron, "The Concept and the Rule of Law," *Georgia Law Review* 43(1), 2008, p. 11; Fukuyama Francis, *State-Building: Governance and World Order in the 21st Century*, Ithaca, NY: Cornell University Press, 2019, p. 59.

[6] Writing of the historical trajectories of the development of the power possessed by states, Michael Mann distinguishes despotic power and infrastructural power, with the

captured a tension in China's responses to the Covid-19 outbreak with the growing abilities for the effective governance to mitigate the Covid-19 spread and its negative socio-economic resulting effects on the one hand, and the predatory deployment of the paternalist campaign-style of governance on the other. On the former issue, community mobilization characterized as grid governance was perceived as an effective measure, despite shortcomings that enable the prevention and control of the Covid-19 pandemic.[7] A whole-government response was perceived as an effective multi-sectoral coordination and whole-of-society measures were seen as successful engagement with different sections of the society.[8] Yet on the other hand, China's responses to the Covid-19 pandemic were viewed as a governance failure, which strengthened, rather than diminished the paternalist campaign-style mode of public health emergency governance.[9] Studies have also criticized the lack of transparency in the Chinese government's coping with this emergency at the early stage.[10]

The vast body of literature presents us with two challenges. First, little attention has been dedicated to the legal and institutional means deployed during different periods of time through China's historical venture into public health emergency management. While it is often recognized that

former denoting "the range of actions which the elite is empowered to undertake without routine, institutionalized negotiation with civil society groups" and the latter referring to "the capacity of the state to actually penetrate civil society, and to implement logistically political decisions throughout the realm". Reflecting on the failure of some states to realize democratization, Francis Fukuyama also identifies enduring divergences of different regimes through three categories of state institutions—i.e., the state, the rule of law, and the accountable government. Studies of China's state capacities have tended to examine mainly extractive and fiscal capacity as well as coercive capacity. Michael Mann, *States, War and Capitalism: Studies in Political Economy*, Oxford: Blackwell, 1988, pp. 5–6; Francis Fukuyama, *The Origins of Political Order: From Prehuman Times to the French Revolution*, p. 16.

[7] *See* Yujun Wei, Zhonghua Ye, Meng Cui & Xiaokun Wei, "Covid-19 Prevention and Control in China: Grid Governance," *Journal of Public Health* 43(1), 2021.

[8] *See* Yan Ning, Ran Ren & Gerad Nkengurutse, "China's Model to Combat the Covid-19 Epidemic: A Public Health Emergency Governance Approach," *Global Health Research and Policy* 5(1), 2020.

[9] *See* Alex Jingwei He, Yuda Shi & Hongdou Liu, "Crisis Governance, Chinese Style: Distinctive Features of China's Response to the Covid-19 Pandemic," *Policy Design and Practice* 3(3), 2020.

[10] Edward Gu & Lantian Li, "Crippled Community Governance and Suppressed Scientific/Professional Communities: A Critical Assessment of Failed Early Warning for the Covid-19 Outbreak in China," *Journal of Chinese Governance* 5(2), 2020.

the party-state organized the whole-of-government and whole-of-society means against pandemics, the question about the differences among the means deployed during patriotic hygiene campaigns, SARS, and the Covid-19 pandemic has not been comprehensively addressed. Second, after the SARS outbreak, the party-state was committed to strengthening the legal and institutional mechanisms in response to public health emergencies. Conversely, much recent literature has investigated how the responses to the public health emergency management indicated a contrast between weak proactive capacity and strong reactive capacity of different parts of the bureaucratic system.[11] Yet this corpus has largely overlooked the intrinsic relationship between the state capacity and the rule of law in the context of the Covid-19 pandemic. After the SARS crisis, it was once commented by scholars that China's failure to reform its political institutions after the SARS outbreak creates worries and fears about whether China has capacities to provide timely and transparent responses to the outbreak of another novel infectious disease. As David Fidler once commented, "China still looms large in any future confrontation with SARS, raising concerns about China's attitude should the virus and disease return. As a group of public health experts observed, '[m]any of the solutions to solve the multifaceted puzzle of SARS and to prevent future epidemics must come from China'".[12] Thus China's responses to the public health emergency outbreaks provide us with a crucial touchstone to examine the rule of law and China's state's capacities, in particular how the legal and institutional means of the public health emergency management have changed over time to cope with unprecedented pandemic challenges, such as the SARS and Covid-19 outbreaks.

This chapter discusses how the Chinese government has exercised emergency power in response to public health emergencies that require decisive executive action and rule of law. Specifically, it examines the legal and institutional means of China's public health emergency management through a historical lens of state power propelled by the emergencies during snail fever patriotic hygiene campaigns, SARS, and the Covid-19 pandemic. It is interested not only in examining the development of

[11] He, Shi & Liu, "Crisis Governance, Chinese Style".

[12] David Fidler, *SARS, Governance and the Globalization of Disease*, London: Palgrave Macmillan, p. 190.

the laws and regulations in the sector of public health emergency management, but analyzing the historical venture of the rule of law in relation to the exercise of state power in response to public health emergencies. After the exploration of the historical trajectories of the public health emergency management system, this chapter also discusses how to understand people's trust in the system during the outbreak of the Covid-19 pandemic.

6.1 Historical Dimension: Patriotic Hygiene Campaigns

In light of the foregoing analysis of a historical dimension to the discussion that follows, a useful historical context for the exploration is the patriotic hygiene campaigns during 1958–1970. As the CCP ascended to power in 1949, China was suffering from disabling infectious diseases. Malaria, plague, cholera, tuberculosis, and smallpox were endemic across the country. Schistosomiasis raged through 105 million people. Highly political patriotic hygiene campaigns were mobilized by the CCP to reduce the pests that transmitted diseases: the mosquitoes that spread malaria, the rodents responsible for plague, and flies that might cause many infectious diseases.

The patriotic hygiene campaigns were developed under "prevention first", which was the official slogan of the post-1949 public health policy.[13] The idea of prevention first was not incorporated to China until the second half of the nineteenth century.[14] The primary considerations for its incorporation were to reduce costs of disease prevention and treatment in the agricultural production sector and to respond to increasing demands of rural populations for access to urban medical facilities.[15] The patriotic hygiene campaigns under the guidance of the "prevention first" policy concentrated on four pests (flies, mosquitoes, rats, and sparrows) and other communicable diseases. Millions of people were mobilized to

[13] C.C. Chen, *Medicine in Rural China: A Personal Account*, Berkeley: University of California Press, 1989, pp. 122–3.

[14] Nianqun Yang, *Remaking the "Patient": The Politics of Space in the Conflict Between Chinese and Western Medicine 1832–1985* [再造 "病人": 中西醫衝突下的空間政治], Beijing: Beijing Renmin University Press, p. 128.

[15] *See* AnElissa Lucas, "Changing Medical Models in China: Organizational Options or Obstacles?" *The China Quarterly* 83 (1980): 461–9.

participate in the campaigns. As characterized by Benjamin Schwartz, the campaign against the "four pests" exemplified the core features of the party-state's endeavor to control the domain of public health:

> [t]he Party's ability to consolidate the enthusiasm and energy of the masses in the war against natural pests and the capacity of the masses to develop simple and yet ingenious methods for dealing with these crucial problems of public health and production could be applied across the board to all sectors of the government.[16]

After such a large number of people were mobilized by the CCP to engage in the campaigns, communicable diseases that had raged in China started to retreat. By the end of 1959, approximately 4.95 million people (accounting for 70% of all the communicated people) were treated and 3.5 million were cured from schistosomiasis suffering.[17]

What, then, might the patriotic hygiene campaigns reveal about the nature of Chinese public health management? First, the policy making and implementation of the patriotic hygiene campaigns were dominated by the CCP, while the professional opinions of the MOH and its institutional mechanisms were applied within a very restricted scope. Mao accused the MOH as "the least healthy"; Mao abandoned the proposal of the MOH on eliminating "four pests" and replaced it with his invention of eradicating the diseases.[18] A central party directive on public health was issued in April 1954, stating that "our leadership work is above all political leadership... Professional work (業務) and technologies have to serve political purposes. Without political leadership there would be no correct or effective professional and technological leadership".[19] To control schistosomiasis, the State Council made schistosomiasis control as "a serious political task". Motivated by the political zeal, Yujiang County of Jiangxi Province claimed to be the first one to have eliminated schistosomiasis.

16 Benjamin Schwartz, "Thoughts on the Late Mao: Between Total Redemption and Utter Frustration", in *The Secrete Speeches of Chairman Mao: From the Hundred Flowers to the Great Leap Forward*, Cambridge: Harvard University Press.

17 Huang, *Governing Health in China*, p. 32.

18 Ibid., 33.

19 Yunbei Xu, "Carrying Out the Great People's Health Work," [開展偉大的人民衛生工作] *Hongqi* 6, 1960, p. 10.

After Mao wrote the poem "Farewell to the God of Plagues", counties and cities started to compete with each other, with 167 of which announced the successful eradication of schistosomiasis. Although professional experts issued advice to extend the time of schistosomiasis from five to ten years, when such a large number of counties and cities claimed quick success in eliminating schistosomiasis, health professionals were criticized heavily. The success of schistosomiasis elimination emboldened Mao to sustain the decision of furthering the campaign against sparrows, even though scientists still had heated debates on whether eliminating sparrows was necessary. In July 1959, while the reduced sparrow population contributed to a plague of locusts, Mao still adhered to the decision of sparrow elimination.[20] In this sense, the professional opinions of the MOH were strongly biased against and placed lower than political leadership of the CCP.

Second, under the CCP's strong leadership, the effective reduction and campaign against the four pests was an embodiment of the Party's mass mobilization—consolidation of the enthusiasm of the masses—while the effective mass mobilization relied on the systematization of linked alternatives and the venture into the domain of public health. Before the patriotic hygiene campaigns were waged widely across China together with the completion of collectivization in rural areas, the Chinese government's penetration into the domain of public health was very limited. Many patriotic hygiene campaigns were waged during 1952–1954. These campaigns were led by the Central Patriotic Hygiene Commission (hereinafter "CPHC"). Similar to the earlier campaigns against the United States bacteriological warfare, a strong message was clearly sent by the party-state that health was no longer an individual responsibility but instead related to national security.[21] Mao personally instructed disease prevention and control. When epidemic control was not emphasized at sub-national level in 1951, Mao said that epidemic control should be viewed as "an important political task".[22] Mao also asked the leaders of the MOH to draft proposals to eradicate schistosomiasis when it was

[20] Huang, *Governing Health in Contemporary China*, p. 34.

[21] On this point, *see* Huang, *Governing Health in Contemporary China*, 28.

[22] Mao Zedong & Zhou Enlai, "Selected Literature of Mao Zedong and Zhou Enlai on Epidemic Control and Medical Care Work," *Literature of Chinese Communist Party* [Dang de Wenxian] 5 (2003), pp. 15–27.

raging southern provinces heavily in 1955.[23] In 1956 Mao even called for "mobilizing the entire party and the entire society to eliminate schistosomiasis".[24] While Mao emphasized the public health concerns and the campaigns, the government's penetration and reach into the entire society was largely constrained by the then state-society relationship structure.

The turning point for the party-state to assert its effective control and reach at the extreme was the completion of communization. The completion of communization in the late 1950s enabled the party-state to extend a web of bureaucratic organs to communities below the county level.[25] In addition, as observed by Huang Yanzhong, public health services could be viewed as incentives for encouraging further collectivization. As put by Huang, "[f]or the Chinese peasants, while the preferred option of individual farming was being closed to them, further collectivization offered them other opportunities and benefits as compensation ".[26] This suggests that the expansion in health and welfare services contributed to the promotion of rural collectivization. Moreover, the provision of the health and welfare services relied on the well-functioning commune system and an increase in agricultural production to provide secure financial and material resources. The rural collectivization and the public health services therefore reinforced each other. This therefore constituted what Tsou Tang calls systematization of linked alternatives.[27]

The systematization of linked alternatives was also reflected in the relationship between the patriotic hygiene campaigns, rural collectivization, and provision of health services. The patriotic hygiene campaigns, as a particular strategy of preventive health, contributed to the increase in agricultural production through reducing pests which ate seeds. The patriotic hygiene campaigns were also predicated upon the well-functioning commune system and the provision of health services. This is because unless peasants had a measure of security in health and food, they would

[23] Huang, *Governing Health in Contemporary China*, p. 28.

[24] Mao Zedong & Zhou Enlai, "Selected Literature of Mao Zedong and Zhou Enlai on Epidemic Control and Medical Care Work," *Dang de wenxian (Literature of Chinese Communist Party)* 5 (2003), pp. 21–2.

[25] Franz Schurmann, *Ideology and Organization in Communist China*, Berkeley, CA: University of California Press.

[26] Huang, *Governing Health in Contemporary China*, p. 30.

[27] Tang Tsou, "Interpreting the Revolution in China: Macrohistory and Micromechanisms," *Modern China* 26(2), 2000, p. 223.

not participate in the campaigns. The process of systematization meant that peasants were obliged and mobilized by "a structure of linked alternatives" rather than an alternative of a single issue to enthusiastically engage in these wide-scale campaigns. As noted by Tsou Tang, "[t]his made it difficult for groups to reject any single preferred alternatives, even when it would hurt their interests, because they would expect benefits from other policies in the structure or would lose those benefits if they rejected the undesired alternative".[28] Thus, the systemization of the linked alternatives not only enabled the CCP's venture into the domain of public health, but contributed to the mass mobilization to engage in the patriotic hygiene campaigns.

Third, the party-state's practice of effectively tackling public health concerns—strong leadership and systemization of linked alternatives—has implications for understanding the form of legitimation. As noted by Perkins and Yusuf,

> The Campaigns of the 1950s legitimized the state's right to supervise sanitary activities in the countryside and to involve itself with what the peasant fed himself and his family and how he reared his children. Layer after layer of privacy, which had shielded peasants from the gaze of the state, was peeled away.[29]

In doing so, the state-party started to penetrate its control over the private ownership and economic activities of peasants. It is suggested that the legitimation of the party-state's venture into the domain of public health is the idea of the mass line. For "mass line" is, as Tsou Tang notes, "[t]o accord with the mass line, leaders in the formulation of policies must go among the masses, listen to their views, systematize them, and take the results back to the masses".[30]

As a method of leadership, the mass line is a means "to ascertain the perceived interests of the masses, a procedure to obtain feedback from them, and a process to assess political realities confronting the party".[31] But this means is different from the basis underpinning a Western liberal democracy. The reason for this is that the concept of the masses is

[28] Ibid.

[29] Perkins & Yusuf, *Rural Development in China*, 1984, p. 137.

[30] Tsou, "Interpreting the Revolution in China," pp. 216–7.

[31] Ibid., 217.

different from the notion of citizenship. The notion of citizenship begins with the view that citizens, as members of the society, are seen as isolated individuals, possessing a series of abstract or legal rights and forming autonomous social groups through exercising these rights; the concept of the masses resides in the view that members are seen as social segments, "possessing not abstract, legal, or civic rights but substantive socioeconomic entitlements".[32] In other words, it is the substantive demands of the masses for socioeconomic justice that incites them to political activism. Thus, the concept of the masses and mass line and the notion of citizenship and liberal democracy denote two different ways of linking the state with society.

The patriotic hygiene campaigns therefore suggest a mobilization-based type of public health campaign that rallied the masses to engage in the war against pests. This type of campaign was launched under the strong party leadership and developed through party-state policies rather than through law and legal institutions. Moreover, the effective implementation of the policies of the campaigns—in terms of achieving the goal of vermin eradication—was underpinned by the notion of the mass line, which reflected the demands of the masses (as segments of society rather than as isolated individuals) for socio-economic justice. With this historical dimension in mind, the following sections identify and discuss the changing nature of public health emergency management, which, it is argued, has implications for understanding the changing nature of the public health emergency management in China.

6.2 SARS Outbreak: China's Turn to Rule of Law in Public Health Emergency Management

This section identifies and discusses legal and institutional developments during and after the SARS outbreak. It explains that the SARS outbreak was an important starting point for the Chinese government to strengthen the rule of law and state capacity in public health emergency management. This analysis revolves around two themes. The first—with reference to the revival of the mass campaign in response to the SARS outbreak—argues that the SARS outbreak revealed the institutional weaknesses of China's

[32] Ibid.

public health emergency management. The second concerns China's post-SARS turn to the rule of law as a new legitimizing weapon to combat infectious disease outbreaks.

In mid-November 2002, a mysterious disease was reported in Foshan, a city southwest of Guangzhou, Guangdong Province. Cases of the unknown disease were subsequently found in the cities of Zhongshan and Heyuan in Guangdong Province. The infectious disease was later identified as severe acute respiratory syndrome ("SARS") caused by a novel coronavirus ("SARS-Cov"). Although the Chinese central government had established a network of epidemic prevention services to report and prevent outbreaks of infectious diseases before the SARS outbreak, the initial responses of the local Guangdong government revealed the institutional weaknesses of public health emergency management in China. It seems certain that the Guangdong government knew about the disease in early January, but it was not until February 3 that the Guangdong Health Department issued a notice on "Prevention and Treatment of Unclear Pneumonia", calling for the disease to be temporarily treated as a type B infectious disease.[33]

A team of experts from the MOH and Guangdong Province was sent to Zhongshan in late January 2003 to prepare an investigation report on this disease. This report was sent to the Guangdong Provincial Health Committee and then to the MOH on January 27, but was classified as top secret and reportedly remained unopened for three days because no one was authorized to read it. When officials were formally authorized to read the document, a bulletin was sent to hospitals in Guangdong province, but most medical professionals were on vacation for the Chinese New Year and few were alerted.[34] A blackout was made on reporting about the disease in government-controlled press, and Guangdong health experts were not allowed to communicate and discuss the disease with experts and health departments of other provinces and Hong Kong.[35] In the meantime, the illness was infecting hundreds of patients, spreading to other parts of China and other 16 countries.[36] Although the MOH was already aware of the disease in late January, it was not until April 3

[33] South China Morning Post, May 17, 2003.

[34] Ibid.

[35] Huang, *Governing Health in Contemporary China*, p. 90.

[36] Pomfret, "China's Slow Reaction to Fast-Moving Illness".

that the Chinese Center for Disease Control and Prevention (hereinafter "CCDC") issued a national bulletin to hospitals on the prevention of the disease from spreading until April 3.[37] Premier Wen Jiabao chaired the first executive meeting of the State Council to discuss disease prevention and control. In the mid-April, SARS was finally listed as a disease to be closely reported on a daily basis according to the Law of Prevention and Treatment of Infectious Diseases ("中華人民共和國傳染病防治法", hereinafter "PTID").[38] This decision was made after at least three months of delay.

A sharp contrast could be witnessed once the decision was made by the Party leaders to intervene in the SARS outbreak. Resources, personnel, and actions of the-whole-of-government and the-whole-of-society were effectively mobilized. On April 23, the SARS Control and Prevention Headquarter of the State Council was established with Vice-Premier Wu Yi as commander-in-chief to coordinate interagency and intergovernmental effects to combat the disease.[39] Similar arrangements were made at each level of government. A fund of two billion *yuan* was created for the prevention and control of SARS on April 23. A SARS hospital which could accommodate 1,200 patients was constructed within one week and started to operate on May 1. On April 20, Beijing Mayor Meng Xuenong and Minister of Health Zhang Wenkang were forced to step down. Nearly 1,000 government officials were disciplined for disobeying central policy instructions. Local governmental offices, shocked by the wide-scale punishment, were forced to jump onto the SARS combat. They sealed off villages, university campuses, set up temperature checkpoints, and quarantined many people. Millions of people were mobilized in Guangdong to clean streets and houses.[40]

Before probing into the differences of the Chinese government's responses toward the two major public health emergency outbreaks, it is crucial to look at the Chinese government's responses before, during, and after the SARS outbreak through institutional and legal establishment. First, while the PTID was drafted by the National People's Congress (hereinafter "NPC") in 1989, the cover-ups and belated responses of the

[37] Huang, *Governing Health in Contemporary China*, p. 90.

[38] Ibid.

[39] Ibid., 125.

[40] Ibid., 92.

local governments of Beijing and Guangdong revealed the institutional weaknesses of the Chinese public health emergency management. The local governments did not follow the procedures laid out by the 1989 PTID and its implementing rules, say, to provide treatment to initial cases, to react quickly to restrict infections as well as to report information timely and accurately to other regions and the public.[41] When SARS spread to Beijing, senior government officials violated the law by hiding information from WHO and misleading the public.[42] The health department ordered hospitals incorrect instructions on dealing with the disease, turning SARS into a global crisis.[43] It was under the Party leadership that the national campaign against SARS was launched and two pieces of laws and regulations were enacted. On May 7, 2003, the State Council issued the Regulation on Handling the Outbreak of Public Health Emergencies ("突發公共衛生事件應急條例", hereinafter "Regulation on Public Health").[44] On May 12, 2003, the Measure on the Prevention and Treatment of Infectious Atypical Pneumonia ("傳染性非典型肺炎防治管理辦法", hereinafter "Measure") was promulgated by the Ministry of Health.[45] The two pieces of laws and regulations mainly addressed emergency information reporting, prevention, and treatment in the way that almost reiterated the requirements of the PTID.[46]

Second, mass mobilization was prevalently adopted during the SARS outbreak. After the adoption of the open-up policy, the Chinese government dismantled communes and reoriented its focus toward costal industrial development. The top-down emphasis and priority of public health management were diminished. During the SARS period, both WHO representatives and the top Chinese political leaders expressed concerns about the spread of disease to rural areas where there was a collapse of

[41] Chenglin Liu, "Regulating SARS in China: Law as an Antidote?" *Washington University Law Review* 4(1), 2005, pp. 84–9.

[42] Ibid., 90–1.

[43] *See* David L. Heymann and Guenael Rodier, "SARS: Lessons from a New Disease," *Learning from SARS: Preparing for the Next Disease Outbreak*, Washington, DC: National Academies Press, 2004.

[44] State Council, Regulation on Handling the Outbreak of Public Health Emergencies ["突發公共衛生事件應急條例"].

[45] Ministry of Health, Measure on the Prevention and Treatment of Infectious Atypical Pneumonia [傳染性非典型肺炎防治管理辦法].

[46] Liu, "Regulating SARS in China," pp. 94–115.

the public health system. After the breakdown of the commune system and the rural cooperative medical system in the late 1970s, healthcare financing was diverted to provinces and local governments. Restricted public finances were allocated to support medical staff salaries at county- and township-level facilities.[47] Some important public health responsibilities and functions, such as surveillance and health education in rural areas, had also been poorly funded over the years. During the SARS outbreak, rural health workers were limited and their training was poorly funded, giving rise to the result that standard infection control practices were not effectively implemented outside urban hospitals.[48] As in the Maoist mobilization-based campaign, the strong party leadership was critical in unifying basic functions and resources of national and local departments; high-level political accountability was created to contain the spread of the virus during the SARS outbreak. Local leaders were mobilized by the political fervor to demonstrate impressive organizational skills in quickly identifying and isolating cases and implementing strict control measures. For example, villages erected barricades to prevent non-residents from entering and to take the temperature of residents. At village gates, people in hazmat suits sprayed disinfectant on floors and passing vehicles. At bus and train stations, airports, and entrances to other public facilities, temporary medical stations were set up to ensure, or at least pretend to ensure, temperature checks for all passersby.[49] These measures had parallels with the patriotic hygiene campaigns. As noted by Huang Yanzhong, "[t]he Maoist 'Patriotic Hygiene Campaign' was also revitalized".[50]

Third, the SARS outbreak also revealed the public distrust in the party-state regime. As one official was reported to have commented, SARS was a "huge shock for the entire party, you can sense this at internal meetings, where the atmosphere has changed and people are expressing criticisms more freely. The SARS epidemic is forcing us to rethink the whole theoretical framework for government that was developed under Jiang

[47] Joan Kaufman, "SARS and China's Health-Care Response: Better to Be Both Red and Expert!" in Arthur Kleinman and James L. Watson, eds., *SARS in China: Prelude to Pandemic?* Stanford, CA: Stanford University Press, 2005, p. 58.

[48] Ibid., 59–60.

[49] Erik Eckholm, "SARS in Beijing: The Unraveling of a Cover-Up," in Arthur Kleinman and James L. Watson, eds., *SARS in China: Prelude to Pandemic?* Stanford, CA: Stanford University Press, 2005, p. 127.

[50] Huang, *Governing Health in Contemporary China*, p. 92.

Zemin".[51] While it was unrealistic to think that the SARS outbreak would lead to fundamental changes in the functioning of the Chinese party-state, it did reveal some challenges that would contribute to increasing public confidence in the party-state. The SARS outbreak "show[ed] that in doing this they will not be able to rely on traditional CCP methods for controlling the country and will be under considerable pressure to find new ways to manage the Chinese polity. It is clear that the forces of globalization will require both a considerable shift in the way that CCP governs the system and the political reform that seeks to make the system not only more transparent but also more accountable".[52] This may be true to understand why reforming the legal system of disease prevention and control became a critical tool for the Chinese government to improve the transparency and accountability of its administration, especially that of local governments. Thus, unlike the patriotic hygiene campaigns, in which, as noted earlier, the Party issued directives necessary to mobilize, say, peasants and lay doctors, the public health strategy of SARS prevention and control is characterized by the political leadership and the legal and institutional arrangements of bureaucratic departments penetrating into the domain of public health.

Law and legal institutions were emphasized by the party-state after the SARS outbreak. After the SARS outbreak, the Chinese government reformed related laws and regulations. The PTID was revised by the NPC on August 28, 2004. The Emergency Response Law ("中華人民共和國突發事件應對法") was also adopted by NPC in 2007. The laws and regulations created a system that defined the entire process of reporting, who to report to, when to report, and what the department should do with the information once it was received.[53] The 2004 PTID

[51] Liu, "Regulating SARS in China," p. 103.

[52] Ibid., 104.

[53] Art 19 of the Regulation on Public Health provides that the Ministry of Health was in command of establishing a public health emergency reporting system. Pursuant to Art 19 of the Regulation on Public Health, when a public health emergency occurs, a provincial government shall report the epidemic information within one hour to the Ministry of Health. Art 20(1) of the Regulation on Public Health requires that medical institutions should report confirmed or suspected cases to local county governments. Art 20.1 further requires that after receiving the information, the local county government should transfer it to higher level of governments within two hours. After finishing the first step of reporting the information to the higher level of governments, the information should move vertically toward higher levels of government and horizontally toward neighboring

contains provisions that double from forty-one to eighteen articles. In addition to emphasizing the vertical information reporting system, Art 35(2) stresses the importance of the horizontal reporting system to neighboring regions. Art 30 requires the government to periodically announce epidemic outbreak situations.

The aforementioned laws and regulations also specified mandatory requirements for treatment, isolation, and quarantine. The revised PTID provides strict regulations on isolation and quarantine. Unlike the 1989 PTID, which required suspected carriers of category A infectious diseases to undergo epidemiological observation at designated places, Art 39(2) of the revised law requires suspected patients to be isolated. The revised PTID also strikes a balance between promoting public health and protecting the individual's right to privacy. Art 12 prohibits hospitals from releasing patients' medical records, with administrative sanctions and criminal liability for violations.

The SARS outbreak also underscored the need to strengthen the institutional arrangements of the disease surveillance network. Before the SARS outbreak, the Chinese central government had established the Epidemic Prevention Services network to prevent outbreaks of infectious diseases. A Center for Disease Control and Prevention (hereinafter "CDC") was created in 2002, so before the SARS outbreak the infrastructure for the public health surveillance and response system was yet established and integrated.

provinces, related government departments, and the public. Art 23(1) of the Regulation on Public Health demands the State Council to disseminate the information promptly to health departments. Art 23(1) further stipulates that the Head of the provinces experiencing an epidemic should release information to neighboring provinces of the outbreak. Art 25 requires reporting the epidemic information to the public; the central government should inform the epidemic information to the public and the local government may be authorized by the central government to announce epidemic outbreaks; and, the announcement should be accurate, up-to-date and comprehensive. In case that any government may not promptly disseminate the epidemic information, the Regulation on Public Health also protects individuals' right to report the outbreaks; Art 24 provides that any individual or unit has the right to report the epidemic outbreaks to government departments, which need to conduct an investigation of the outbreaks. Art 21 prescribes that any individual or unit should not delay, conceal, or falsely report the outbreak information. As further required by Art 45, the head of the department ought to take the liability for the failure to report. The sanctions provided by this article include administrative penalties, such as demotion to a lower rank, and criminal charges. The interpretations of the Supreme Court and Procuratorate specify critical charges against persons who fail to report crucial information, which may further lead to massive spreads of the disease.

The Chinese system was modeled on the Centers for Disease Control and Prevention in the United States. The National CDC, like the former Chinese Academy of Preventive Medicine, was under the control of the MOH and served to strengthen communication among epidemic prevention stations. It was mandated to better inform health policy by collecting health information, strengthening emergency response mechanisms, and improving preventive health services. It was specifically responsible for clinical preventive health research, epidemiological research, formulation of prevention and control plans, and management of environmental and health policies.[54] Local CDCs operating at the regional, municipal, and district levels within health departments and bureaus were also coordinated by the MOH. With the disease reporting system in place, county-level cases were reported by mail through the municipal CDC, provincial CDC, and eventually the national CDC.[55]

The SARS outbreak revealed the weakness of this epidemic surveillance system. As Gao Qiang, the Executive-Vice-Minister of Health admitted, "a weak epidemic surveillance system was among the major causes of the SARS outbreak in 2003".[56] Following the SARS outbreak, a new Internet-based disease reporting system was launched in 2004 to replace the previous postal system, making it easier for hospitals and health centers to report suspected cases of disease directly to the MOH and the national CDC in a timely manner. Health emergency response offices were also established at the provincial and city levels by 2008. When an infectious disease is laboratory confirmed and/or clinically diagnosed, cases must be reported to the national CDC. With the Internet-based disease reporting system, the average time between the identification of a disease case and the reporting of the case to the national CDC was reduced from 29 days to less than 2 hours for all category A diseases and specified category B diseases, and 24 hours for all category B unspecified diseases.[57] After its reorganization in 2004, CDC was focused on

[54] *See* Jonathan Schwartz, R. Gregory Evans & Sarah Greenberg, "Evolution of Health Provision in PreSars China," *China Review*, 2007, p. 92.

[55] Peng Jia & Shujuan Yang, "China Needs a National Intelligent Syndromic Surveillance System," *Nature Medicine* 26(7), 2020, p. 990.

[56] Gao Qiang, "Executive Vice Minister of Health Gao Qiang and Others Answer Questions on the Prevention and Treatment of SARS" [衛生部常務副部長高強等就非典防治情況答問], http://news.enorth.com.cn/system/2003/04/21/000547490.shtml.

[57] Ibid.

addressing emerging infectious disease threats by coordinating prevention and control efforts and providing technical assistance to local and regional EPS, which became CDC offices.[58] More generally, the SARS outbreak was a turning point for the Chinese government in emphasizing the rule of law and transparency. In the same year as the SARS outbreak, there were widespread calls for and commitments to greater transparency. In 2004, the constitution was amended to recognize the protection of human rights and private property.[59] Apart from the Emergency Response Law, which was enacted in 2007, there were five types of emergency events regulated by the law—including wars, natural disasters, accidents and catastrophes, public health events, and social security events.[60]

[58] Chen Zhuo, "COVID-19 and the Case for Empowering China's CDC," *Sixth Tone*, March 28, 2020.

[59] Benjamin Liebman, "Legal Reform: China's Law-Stability Paradox," *Daedalus* 143 (2), 2014, p. 98.

[60] The laws that adjust the five types of emergency events are accordingly divided into three categories: war law (戰爭法), emergency law (緊急狀態法), and emergency response law (應急狀態法). A war is regulated by statutes related to war, including the National Defense Law (國防法), Military Service Law (兵役法), National Defense Mobilization Law (國防動員法), etc. An emergency is regulated by a set of statutes that adjust the state of emergency (緊急狀態), including the Martial Law (戒嚴法). An emergency response is regulated by a category of statutes that adjust the state of emergency incidents (突發事件). This category of statutes is created in accordance with the Constitution. It is composed of the Emergency Response Law, Infectious Disease Prevention Law, Earthquake Prevention and Disaster Mitigation Law, Flood Prevention Law, Safety Production Law, Emergency Regulations on Public Health Emergencies, Nuclear Power Plant Emergency Management Regulations, etc. Four types of emergency incidents are regulated by the Emergency Response Law—including, natural disasters, accidents, public health events, and social security events. According to the degree of social damage and its negative effects, the Emergency Response Law categorizes emergency incidents into four levels—including, especially serious incidents, serious incidents, large incidents, and ordinary incidents. The Emergency Response Law specifies the creation of epistemic and power-creating functions at the central level, and it also clarifies the parallel power-creating function at the local level. Arts 8 and 9 of the Emergency Response Law create executive's emergency powers to decide the outbreak of emergency incidents and to deploy responses to the incidents. The State Council under the leadership of the Premier is authorized to recognize the fact of a serious emergency incident outbreak, but it is unclear which administrative organ is authorized to recognize the outbreak of the other three types of emergency incidents. After the recognition of the fact of an emergency incident, the State Council is permitted to deploy responses to an especially serious emergency incident, and a state emergency response command body is permitted to assume the duty to respond to the emergency incident. At the local level, an emergency response command body is permitted to lead

Thus, this section has argued that the SARS outbreak marked China's turn to the rule of law through its venture into public health management, although this turn was probably not something actively chosen by the partial state, but an inevitable choice to overcome the challenge to its regime legitimacy. The previous laws and regulations constituted a legal system for public health emergency management; however, as will be explained in the following section, the institutional framework for public health emergency management developed after the SARS outbreak remained fragmented, foreshadowing the chaos of China's early struggle with the Covid-19 pandemic.

6.3 COVID-19 Pandemic: Penetration of the Rule of Law into Public Health Emergency Management

It was noted earlier that the SARS outbreak marked the beginning of China's turn to the rule of law in public health emergency management. Using the example of China's responses to the Covid-19 outbreak, this section aims to illustrate that while the implementation of laws and regulations was sluggish in the early stages of the outbreak, the laws and regulations, legal administration, and judicial practices in the later stages witnessed further penetration of the rule of law in the public health emergency management.

In December 2019, another mysterious disease was reportedly found in a hospital in the city of Wuhan, the capital of Hubei province. The cause of the pneumonia was later determined to be a new coronavirus known as SARS-CoV-2. As noted above, the extremely painful lessons learned from the delayed response to the SARS outbreak had enabled the Chinese government to reform outdated legislation and establish a new Internet reporting mechanism. Despite these efforts, implementation of the laws and regulations on reporting and information sharing was still sluggish in the early stages of the Covid-19 outbreak.

The local governments of Wuhan and Hubei were criticized for their delayed early warning. The first case of this "unknown pneumonia" was reported to be found on 8 December 2020. Despite the increasingly huge

and coordinate the activities of different local government departments. In addition, Art 12 stipulates that the property of entities and individuals may be requisitioned, but once the emergency subsides and the normal life resumes, ordinary legal and political processes will be returned and the requisitioned property must be returned timely.

number of suspicious cases, whistleblowers (including Dr. Li Wenliang) failed to issue early warnings for the public or to take systematic precautionary actions until the evidence of human-to-human was confirmed on 20 January 2020.[61] The widespread online discussions were even suppressed by secret directives issued by the Cyberspace Administration of China.[62] It was believed that "the most favorable time for containing the spread of the virus was lost amidst the rapid large-scale flow of travelers to and from Wuhan during China's busiest spring festival season".[63] On January 23, the critical decision was made to seal off Wuhan. As the disease spread to Hong Kong and other provinces across China, all 31 provinces in China initiated the highest level of public health emergency response by January 29.[64]

While many factors were believed to contribute to the delayed early warnings made by the local departments,[65] the inconsistencies between the main laws on public health emergency management and institutional fragmentation were important. The Emergency Response Law establishes a bottom-up emergency reporting system.[66] For example, regarding who is responsible for informing the public about the outbreak of an unknown disease, according to the Emergency Response Law, the county government is not only responsible for reporting to higher levels of government, but is also required to release emergency information to the public on a timely and regular basis. In contrast, the 2013 PCID adopts a top-down management system. According to the 2013 PCID, the MOH

[61] Gu & Li, "Crippled Community Governance and Suppressed Scientific/Professional Communities".

[62] Raymond Zhong, Paul Mozur and Aaron Krolik, "Leaked Documents Show How China's Army of Paid Internet Trolls Helped Censor the Coronavirus," *ProPublica & New York Times*, https://www.propublica.org/article/leaked-documents-show-how-chinas-army-of-paid-internet-trolls-helped-censor-the-coronavirus.

[63] He, Shi & Liu, "Crisis Governance, Chinese Style," p. 243.

[64] Caixin, "31 Provinces of China initiated level-one response o public health emergency" [中國內地 31 省份全部啓動突發公共衛生事件一級回應], http://china.caixin.com/2020-01-29/101509411.html.

[65] For instance, insufficient autonomy of the scientific communities was identified as a major factor contributing to the failed implementation of the early warning mechanism. See Gu & Li, "Crippled Community Governance and Suppressed Scientific/Professional Communities".

[66] Art 7 of the Emergency Response Law stipulates that the government at the county level is responsible for responding to an emergency accident.

(now the National Health and Family Planning Commission, hereinafter "NHFPC") is mandated to regularly and timely release information on the nationwide epidemic situations of infectious diseases to the public, and it is also allowed to authorize the provincial-level health departments to release information on the epidemic situations of infectious diseases in their administrative regions. Thus, the 2013 PCID does not require either city-level or county-level health departments to report the incidence of infectious diseases to the public. The inconsistency between the two statutes caused problems in implementation. As a result, it was unclear who had the power and authority to release emergency outbreak information, which may explain why the local governments of Wuhan and Hubei did not release information to the public about the outbreak of an unknown disease.

In addition to the aforementioned inconsistencies between the key laws and regulations governing public health emergency management, the institutional fragmentation of the *tiao-kuai* also contributed to the confusing situation. When local CDCs collected information, many of them tended to report only to the county health department rather than to the municipal or provincial CDCs.[67] The health departments at the county level were controlled by the county governments, and therefore officials at the county health bureaus had enormous disincentives when reporting disease information up the administrative ladder, such as threats to their personal advancement within the government and Party should they make negative reports.[68] Moreover, the CCDC and the local CDCs of Wuhan failed to report the cases of unknown etiology, while other members of the Chinese epidemiological community, such as both public and private research organizations, were not allowed to conduct virological testing and studies at the early stage of the Covid-19 outbreak.[69] The malfunction of the internet direct reporting system at this stage

[67] Yuanli Liu, "China's Public Health-Care System: Facing the Challenges," *Bulletin of the World Health Organization* 82(7), 2004, pp. 532–8; Central Intelligence Agency, "SARS: Lesson from the First Epidemic of the 21st Century," p. 7; Robert Beaglehole & Ruth Bonita, "Public Health Themes: Historical and Contemporary," *Public Health at the Crossroads*, Cambridge: Cambridge University Press, 1997, p. 45.

[68] Yuanli Liu, "China's Public Health-Care System: Facing the Challenges," *Bulletin of the World Health Organization* 82(7), 2004, p. 533.

[69] Gu & Li, "Crippled Community Governance and Suppressed Scientific/Professional Communities," p. 164.

was another factor further complicating the problem.[70] In this sense, even if the statutes and regulations specified the appropriate responses of the public health emergency management and the reporting procedure, the institutional structure in which the statute was implemented still compromised their legal effects.

Similar to what happened during the SARS outbreak, after the whole country went into emergency mode, effective measures were quickly taken with enormous resources and a high degree of social control. At the legislative level, Covid-19 was included among the Type B infectious diseases specified in the 2013 Law on the Prevention and Control of Infectious Diseases. Measures for the prevention and control of Type A infectious diseases were included in the management of infectious diseases under quarantine, as stipulated in the Frontier Health and Quarantine Law. On January 20, Chairman Xi Jinping made important instructions on the prevention and control of the pandemic, emphasizing the priority of people's lives and health.[71] At various stages of the Covid-19 pandemic, Chairman Xi made response demands at high-level meetings to bring together officials of different ministerial and hierarchical systems.[72] The Central Leading Group for Prevention and Control of Covid-19 (hereinafter "CLG"), headed by Premier Li Keqiang and composed of senior political members of the CCP Politburo and the State Council, was established to coordinate inter-ministerial activities and mobilize personnel, material, and financial resources. It issued "directives [that] were considered as uncompromisable political tasks to be fulfilled by participants".[73] The Central Steering Group for the Prevention and Control of Covid-19 (hereinafter "CSG"), composed of 11 ministerial-level cadres, was also established as the CLG's representative to oversee the frontline control of the Covid-19 outbreak in Hubei Province.[74]

[70] Wei, Furong, Meng Du, & Yifan Zhang, "Wuhan Yiqing Chuqi, Wangluo Zhibao Xitong Weihe Shiling" [武漢疫情初期, 網路直報系統為何失靈], Phoenix New Media, https://news.ifeng.com/c/7uqH6A5PWt7.

[71] Xinhua News, "Xi Focus: Chronicle of Xi's Leadership in China's War Against Coronavirus," http://www.xinhuanet.com/english/2020-09/07/c_139349538.htm.

[72] Ibid.

[73] He, Shi & Liu, "Crisis Governance, Chinese Style," 246.

[74] Sohu News, "Central Leadership Group for the First Time Disclosed! 11 Ministerial-Level Cadres in Hubei Front-Line Coordination and Command" [中央領導組首次披露! 11位部級幹部在湖北一線協調指揮], https://www.sohu.com/a/378422340_120053683.

Parallel epidemic prevention and control headquarters were also established in regions across China to coordinate the activities of lower-level commissions and ministries.

Under the leadership of the CLG, functional boundaries between commissions and ministries, as well as geographical boundaries between provinces, were overcome. For example, the National Health Commission (hereinafter "NHC"), the military, the Ministry of Transportation, the Ministry of Industry and Information Technology, the Ministry of Education, the Supreme Court, and other state organs, as well as their local departments, were all mobilized to fight Covid-19.[75] Enormous administrative regulations were issued by the central-level commissions and ministries. 536 documents were issued as Covid-19 countermeasure-related documents released by the related departments (see Chart 3.1).[76] On the interpretative level, the Supreme People's Court issued notices and announcements. They included, in the area of civil, commercial, and economic law, intellectual property tribunal on the arrangements for legal proceedings and litigation services,[77] intellectual property tribunal on the arrangement for online case filing and mailing of case-filing materials,[78] the enforcement work,[79] online litigation,[80] judicial departments

[75] Jacques DeLisle & Kui Shen, "China's Response to COVID-19," *Administrative Law Review* 73(1), 2021, p. 44.

[76] 536 documents on infectious disease prevention and control were issued by the central government departments between January 24, 2020 and January 1, 2021. Source: Compiled by the author from the feature column in PKULaw (access January 4, 2021).

[77] Announcement of the Intellectual Property Tribunal of the Supreme People's Court on the Arrangements for Legal Proceedings and Litigation Services during the Prevention and Control of the Covid-19 Outbreak, "最高人民法院智慧財產權法庭關於疫情防控期間訴訟活動, 訴訟服務工作安排的公告," January 29, 2020.

[78] Announcement of the Intellectual Property Tribunal of the Supreme People's Court on Matters concerning Online Case Filing and Mailing of Case-filing Materials during the Prevention and Control of the Covid-19 Outbreak, "最高人民法院智慧財產權法庭關於新型冠狀病毒感染的肺炎疫情防控期間網上立案、郵寄立案事宜的公告," January 29, 2020.

[79] Notice by the Enforcement Bureau of the Supreme People's Court of Matters concerning Effectively Conducting the Enforcement Work during the Period of Prevention and Control of the Outbreak of Novel Coronavirus Pneumonia, "最高人民法院執行局關於做好防控新型冠狀病毒肺炎疫情期間執行工作相關事項的通知," January 30, 2020.

[80] Notice by the Supreme People's Court of Strengthening and Regulating the Online Litigation Work During the Period of Prevention and Control of the Covid-19 Outbreak, "最高人民法院關於新冠肺炎疫情防控期間加強和規範線上訴訟工作的通知," February 14, 2020.

leally ensuring the resumption of work and production,[81] three notices on hearing civil cases,[82] and travel contract disputes resolution.[83] Legal mechanism that was allowed or encouraged by the Chinese government to check government performance was administrative litigation and mass tort suits against private and public entities (Table 6.1).[84]

Similar to what happened during the SARS outbreak, the "absorb" method was taken during the Covid-19 pandemic.[85] This method was consistent with the requirements of Art 50 of the PCID. All Covid-19 patients were required to receive treatment at hospitals where they were in the first place admitted. Hospitals were also required to provide patients with free treatments.[86] At the initial stage of the Covid-19 outbreak, the

[81] Notice by the CPC Political and Legislative Affairs Committee, the Supreme People's Court, and the Supreme People's Procuratorate of Issuing the Opinions on Procuratorial, Judicial and Public Security Departments Legally Ensuring the Resumption of Work and Production during the Epidemic Prevention and Control, "中共中央政法委員會, 最高人民法院, 最高人民檢察院等關於印發《關於政法機關依法保障疫情防控期間復工複產的意見》的通知", February 25, 2020.

[82] Notice by the Supreme People's Court of Issuing the Guiding Opinions (Part I) on Several Issues of Properly Hearing Civil Cases concerning the COVID-19 Pandemic, "最高人民法院印發《關於依法妥善審理涉新冠肺炎疫情民事案件若干問題的指導意見 (一)》"; Notice by the Supreme People's Court of Issuing the Guiding Opinions (Part II) on Several Issues of Properly Hearing Civil Cases concerning the COVID-19 Pandemic, "最高人民法院印發《關於依法妥善審理涉新冠肺炎疫情民事案件若干問題的指導意見 (二)》"; Notice by the Supreme People's Court of Issuing the Guiding Opinions (Part III) on Several Issues of Properly Hearing Civil Cases concerning the COVID-19 Pandemic, "最高人民法院印發《關於依法妥善審理涉新冠肺炎疫情民事案件若干問題的指導意見 (三)》".

[83] Notice by the Supreme People's Court, the Ministry of Justice, and the Ministry of Culture and Tourism of Legally and Properly Resolving Travel Contract Disputes involving the COVID-19 Pandemic, "最高人民法院, 司法部, 文化和旅遊部關於依法妥善處理涉疫情旅遊合同糾紛有關問題的通知".

[84] For instance, the Supreme People's Procuratorate published "typical cases of public interest litigation on wildlife protection by procuratorial organs" ("檢察機關野生動物保護公益訴訟典型案例") on February 28, 2020.

[85] National Health Commission, Notice on the issuance of the recent work program for the prevention and control of pneumonia with novel coronavirus infection [關於印發近期防控新型冠狀病毒感染的肺炎工作方案的通知], http://www.nhc.gov.cn/xcs/zhengcwj/202001/808bbf75e5ce415aa19f74c78ddc653f.shtml.

[86] People's Daily Online, "National Health Insurance Bureau: People-Centered, Effective Protection of Patients' Medical Costs" [國家醫保局: 以人民為中心, 切實保障患者醫療費用], http://society.people.com.cn/n1/2020/0329/c1008-31652667.html.

Table 6.1 Data collected from PKULaw

National Health Commission (衛生健康委員會)	64
Ministry of Transport (交通運輸部)	53
Ministry of Finance (財政部)	48
Ministry of Civil Affairs(民政部)	34
Ministry of Commerce(商務部)	33
Ministry of Human Resource and Social Security(人力資源和社會保障部)	30
Ministry of Education(教育部)	23
State Administration for Market Regulation (國家市場監督管理總局)	21
State Taxation Administration (國家稅務總局)	18
National Development and Reform Commission(國家發展和改革委員會)	17
Ministry of Agriculture and Rural Affairs(農業農村部)	16
Ministry of Housing and Urban and Rural Development(住房和城鄉建設部)	14
Others	204

"absorb" requirement was not effectively implemented in Wuhan.[87] Due to the lack of beds and isolation points, suspected and mild patients were required to receive isolation at home. While this strategy might restrict the spread of infections to the outside world, the homes of suspected and mild patients became sources of infections. In order to impede the spread of infection during the pandemic, the Chinese government demonstrated outstanding mobilizational capacity in extracting enormous human and material resources. Online medical consultation was provided by hospitals soon after the outbreak. When people had access to professional

[87] Sohu News, Wuhan to Promote the Policy "All Patients Should Be Collected", How to Do? What Is the Difficulty? [武漢推進 "應收盡收", 如何做? 難在哪?], https://www.sohu.com/a/371492993_118392.

medical guidance and consultation through mobile devices or computers, their anxiety and panic could be reduced during the initial stage of the pandemic outbreak.[88]

Three conditions were crucial to realize the extractive capacity of the Chinese government. First, the Chinese government had the capacity to steer massive resources from military and civilian subordinates. The People's Liberation Amy (hereinafter "PLA"), for instance, has played an important role in sending 4,000 military health workers and abundant medical equipment and supplies to Wuhan. One of the two shelter hospitals was also controlled by military medical teams.[89] Second, the Chinese government had a favorable advantage due to the huge amount of state-owned enterprises (hereinafter "SOE") as a solid economic foundation for resource mobilization. Given that SOEs were subject to soft budget constraints and dominate strategic industries, large SOEs could provide massive equipment and supplies to the Covid-19 combat.[90] Third, the extractive capacity through taxation was another factor guaranteeing the revenue availability of the Chinese government. As Joseph Schumpeter characterizes the modern state as a "tax state",[91] the extractive capacity through taxation provides the economic foundation for other sate capacities. In accordance with the notices issued by the Ministry of National Medical Insurance, hospitals should provide Covid-19 patients with free treatment.[92] To ensure that patients could be admitted and to dispel the worry of hospitals about budget constraints, the Ministry of National Medical Insurance timely adjusted the total budget indicators of designated hospitals, and spared budgets for medical expenses. In order to relieve the pressure on hospitals to advance funds, medical insurance

[88] Meijun Shu & Jiarui Li, "Health Digital Technology in COVID-19 Pandemic: Experience from China," *BMJ Innovations* 6(4), 2020.

[89] He, Shi & Liu, "Crisis Governance, Chinese Style," p. 249.

[90] Ibid.

[91] Richard Swedberg, ed., *Joseph A. Schumpeter: The Economics and Sociology of Capitalism*, Princeton University Press, 2020.

[92] CNR News, "Behind the 17,000 *Yuan* Per Capita Medical Cost of Covid-19 Patients: A People-Centered Health Insurance System" [新冠肺炎患者人均醫療費用 1.7 萬元背後: 以人民為中心的醫保制度], http://news.cnr.cn/native/gd/20200331/t20200331_525036902.shtml.

agencies also prepared special funds for patient treatment, and the public finance also supported the expenses paid by patients.[93]

Other medical countermeasures included testing and screening[94] as well as vaccination. The restricted nucleic acid reagent testing kits at the early stage of the outbreak restricted the capacities of hospitals to receive patients. Due to the extremely insufficient supply of nucleic acid reagent testing kits, many suspected patients had to wait for tests. Without receiving tests, they could not be admitted into designated hospitals, leading to the potential of further spread.[95] On February 5, the NHC included CT images as another clinical diagnostic criterion by releasing the fifth version of the "New Coronavirus Infection Pneumonia Diagnosis Program"; however, this new diagnostic standard did not apply to Hubei. It was until February 12 that this standard was not applicable in Hubei.[96] When the domestic Covid-19 transmission had been basically controlled, the detection capacity was accelerated to prevent imported infections. Since April 22, 2020, large-scale nucleic acid testing was adopted to prevent the pandemic from rebounding.[97] Vaccines have been provided for patients to immunize the population against the disease. The provision of vaccines is free to citizens in China. The Chinese plan to achieve community immunity takes two steps: the first step targets at key populations, including those who are engaged in the work with a high occupational explosion risk and those who are to work and study abroad in medium and high-risk countries; and the second step is to gradually

[93] "National Health Insurance Bureau: People-Centered, Effective Protection of Patients' Medical Costs," http://www.xinhuanet.com/politics/2020-03/29/c_1125784154.htm.

[94] By testing, it means "a clinical procedure that determines the presence or absence of disease, or its precursor, in an individual patient"; by screening, it refers to "the systematic application of a medical test to a defined population". Lawrence O. Gostin & Lindsay F. Wiley, *Public Health Law: Power, Duty, Restraint*, Berkeley: University of California Press, 2016, p. 365.

[95] Southern Weekly, "Wuhan 'Collection as Much as Possible' Where Is the Difficulty" ["武漢 '應收盡收' 難在何處"], http://www.infzm.com/contents/177054.

[96] Ibid.

[97] Central Commission for Discipline Inspection of the Communist Party of China, "The Central Committee of the Communist Party of China: To Carry Out Large-Scale Nucleic Acid and Antibody Testing," http://www.ccdi.gov.cn/toutiao/202004/t20200424_216055.html.

expand the scope of those receiving vaccines and to realize the objective of community immunity.[98]

Apart from the primary and secondary medical countermeasures, subtle tactics were adopted to encourage citizens to follow hygiene requirements. Simply putting hand sanitizer dispensers or tissues nearby increased chances that people used them before entering a building, even when people carried their own tissues and sanitizers. Standing spots were also served as subtle reminders to keep two meters from others. While these measures could have been implemented without labeled standing spots, the standing spots removed the mental efforts for people to have to figure out how far to stand from each other.

Since the Covid-19 pandemic took place in a digital age, means of digital technology were widely deployed to enable the party-state to "see" the society.[99] Intelligence tracking, mass surveillance, and large data technology were adopted for pandemic predication and alerts, tracing and tracking of infected patients, identifying pharmacological treatments, resource allocations within the health system, etc.[100] Chinese citizens were encouraged to install the QR code system, allowing governmental authorities to inspect whether they had been exposed to the virus. This system, enabled by a nationwide telecom data analysis platform under the Ministry of Information Industry Technology, allowed three major telecom carriers of China (China Mobile, China Telecom, and China Unicom) to provide a tracking record of citizens' locations in the past 15 or 30 days.[101] Thus, given that almost half of the Chinese citizens have now possessed smart phones and the Chinese government has adopted the sophisticated means of digital technology to make the

[98] New Hunan, "New Crown Vaccination Program Determined! Health Commission: National Vaccination in a Two-Step Program" [新冠疫苗接種方案確定! 衛健委: 全國接種疫苗分兩步方案], https://hunan.voc.com.cn/xhn/article/202012/202012191037322076.html.

[99] *See* James Scott, *Seeing Like a State: How Certain Schemes to Improve the Human Condition Have Failed*, New Haven, CT: Yale University Press, 1998.

[100] Jun Wu, Jian Wang, Stephen Nicholas, et al. "Application of Big Data Technology for COVID-19 Prevention and Control in China: Lessons and Recommendations," *Journal of Medical Internet Research* 22(10), 2020.

[101] Lydia Khalil, "Digital Authoritarianism, China and Covid," *Lowy Institute Analysis*, https://www.lowyinstitute.org/publications/digital-authoritarianism-china-and-covid; https://www.nortonrosefulbright.com/en-cn/knowledge/publications/d7a9a296/contact-tracing-apps-a-new-world-for-data-privacy.

society legible and predictable.[102] From SARS to Covid-19, China's public health institutions have been evolving from a Panopticon—a static model of centralized, one-way surveillance—into what Manuel DeLanda has termed as Panspectron.[103] According to DeLanda,

> Instead of positioning some human bodies around a central sensor, a multiplicity of sensors is deployed around all bodies: its antenna farms, spy satellites and cable-traffic intercepts feed into its computers all the information that can be gathered. [...] The Panspectron does not merely select certain bodies and certain (visual) data about them. Rather, it compiles information about all the same time, using computers to select the segments of data relevant to its surveillance task.[104]

The digital tools of contact tracing were different from the traditional manual tracing method deployed during the SARS outbreak. For instance, for contact tracing of cases of AIDS, HIV-related illness or HIV infection, traditional manual tracing method requires patients and suspected patients to report to the health department of information regarding known contacts; the health department then notified patients of potential exposure by phone calls or in person. By contrast, the digital applications for contact tracing allow the Chinese government to monitor, guide, and control people's behaviors in a non-coercive manner. Moreover, these digital measures for contact tracing and mobility restrictions were mostly provided by private technology companies instead of the government organs, because these measures relied on massive computing and data capacities.[105]

In October 2020 after recognizing the inconsistencies of the provisions within the 2013 PCID and with other related ones stipulated in

[102] Ibid.

[103] As observed by Rogier Creemers, China's cyberspace is observed to be "evolving from a Panopticon, a static model of centralized, one-way observation and surveillance, into what Manuel DeLanda has termed as a Panspectron". Rogier Creemers, "Cyber China: Upgrading Propaganda, Public Opinion Work and Social Management for the Twenty-First Century," *Journal of Contemporary China* 26, 2017, p. 88.

[104] Manuel Delanda, *War in the Age of Intelligent Machines*, New York: Swerwe Editions, 1991, pp. 205–6.

[105] Mengji Chen, Shan Xu, Lewis Husain & Gauden Galea, "Digital Health Interventions for Covid-19 in China: A Retrospective Analysis," *Intelligent Medicine* 1(1), 2021, p. 33.

other statutes and regulations, the Notice of Consultation on the PCID was issued. The revision revolved around two central issues. The first was to expand the scope of governmental entities to include the CDC at the county level to issue early warning of infectious diseases in a timely manner, which aimed to deal with the conflicts between the provisions of the 2013 PCID and the Law on Emergency Response. The revised version of the PCID requires the health department at or above the county level to promptly and accurately release information regarding the outbreak of an infectious disease of the administrative region, the name of the infectious disease, the scope of the epidemic spread, the numbers of confirmed and suspected cases and deaths of the infectious disease to the public.[106] The revised version of the PCID would thus eliminate the inconsistency with the Law on Emergency Response, clarifying the reporting procedures and improving the quality of the PCID.

The second major revision is to provide for detailed responses respectively to the three types of infectious diseases. On the basis of the three types of notifiable infectious diseases—Types A, B and C, Art 38 of the revised statute adds "an unexplained cluster disease with epidemiological characteristics of an infectious disease". Art 38 also prescribes that when the disease prevention and control agency receives a report on the epidemic situation of a Type A infectious disease or an unexplained cluster disease with epidemiological characteristics of an infectious disease and an outbreak of other infectious diseases, it shall complete the epidemic information verification and report to the local health authority within 2 hours. The report shall be immediately reported to the local people's government by the local health department, and to the health department at a higher level and the health department under the State Council.[107] The revised provisions regarding the procedures will, then, be consistent with those prescribed in the Regulation on Infectious Disease Information Reporting Management, as an administrative regulation issued by the

[106] Art 43 stipulates that when infectious diseases break out or spread across provinces, autonomous regions, and municipalities directly under the Central Government, the health authority of the State Council is responsible for releasing the epidemic information. The standards for the publication of infectious disease epidemic information shall be formulated by the health authority of the State Council.

[107] "The National Health Commission on the Law on the Prevention and Control of Infectious Diseases" [國家衛生健康網委關於《中華人民共和國傳染病防治法》(修訂草案徵求意見稿) 公開徵求意見的通知], http://www.nhc.gov.cn/fzs/s3577/202010/330ecbd72c3940408c3e5a49e8651343.shtml.

NHFPC of a lower status than the PCID. Through clarifying the classification of the types of infectious diseases, the revision will improve the efficiency of the prevention and control mechanisms of infectious diseases.

Moreover, when China was restructuring CDC in 2004, it was also revising the notifiable disease diagnostic criteria and launching a national centralized web-based reporting system. The Infectious Disease Automatize-Alert and Response System (hereinafter "CIDARS") and the Notifiable Infectious Disease Reporting Information System (hereinafter "NIDRIS") were arranged to focus on already-designated infectious diseases, two new surveillance systems—the Sentinel Influenza-like Illness (hereinafter "ILI") and the Pneumonia of Unexplained Etiology (hereinafter "PUE")—were built after the SARS outbreak. Healthcare facilities were required to report cases "who have a clinical diagnosis of pneumonia with an unknown causative pathogen and whose disease meets the five criteria of pneumonia diagnosis to the PUE system".[108] Once cases are registered under NIDRIS, the data of the cases are further analyzed as type I infectious diseases in CIDARS.[109] A National Administration of Disease Prevention and Control, a vice-ministerial-level agency under the NHC, was inaugurated on May 13, 2021. The roles and functions of the disease prevention and control agencies will be expanded to encompass a comprehensive safeguarding and promotion of the health of the population. While it remains unclear how the local and regional institutions will be reformed it seems clear that a tiered network of public health emergency management teams will be set up and related mechanisms will be built to coordinate their work.[110]

[108] Jennifer Bouey, "China's Health System Reform and Global Health Strategy in the Context of COVID-19," *Rand*, 2020, p. 7.

[109] Ibid.

[110] Xinhua, "China Focus: China Inaugurates National Administration of Disease Prevention and Control," http://www.xinhuanet.com/english/2021-05/13/c_139943875.htm; 21st Century Business Herald, "China's CDC System "Epidemic" Change: Upgrading, Integration, Synergy, Sinking" [中國疾控體系 "疫" 變: 升格, 整合, 協同, 下沉], https://m.21jingji.com/article/20210512/846b0b8a1047ae55bb76280fe9a019bb.html.

6.4 People's Trust in the Public Health Management System During the Covid-19 Pandemic

This chapter began with an exploration of the historical legacy of patriotic hygiene campaigns in China. It sought to show that despite the state's strong despotic power, the capacity of the state to penetrate into the public health management sector was restricted. It also examined China's responses to the SARS outbreak and the subsequent legal development. It argued that the SARS outbreak marked the state's beginning of its move on the trajectory of the rule of law in the public health emergency management sector. This section also discusses the changes of people's trust in the healthcare system during the Covid-19 pandemic.

One way to approach this question is to examine the state capacity of the CCP government in financing efforts to cope with the Covid-19 pandemic. Although the CCP government increased its state capacity in response to public health emergencies, it also demonstrated significant limitations in healthcare financing, which could lead to a decline in patient confidence and trust in public hospitals. During the Covid-19 pandemic, the ability of the medical insurance system to effectively respond to the health needs of the local population is often questioned. Since the outbreak of the Covid-19 pandemic, physicians have played a critical role in containment, diagnosis, and treatment. Their commitment to treatment has presented a selfless and heroic figure of benevolent saviors that has inspired patient trust. In contrast, the role of China's social health insurance system has been criticized for its lack of sustainability.[111] A document called the Opinions on Deepening Healthcare Insurance System Reform (hereinafter "Opinions") was issued by the CPC central committee and the State Council on 25 February 2020.[112] The Opinions outline the reform objectives to be reached respectively by 2025 and 2030, the measures to improve the security and sustainability of the social healthcare insurance system, and the principles to enhance the competence of the healthcare insurance reform. While the Opinions

[111] Sun, Shuangyi, Zhen Xie, Keting Yu, Bingqian Jiang, Siwei Zheng, & Xiaoting Pan, "COVID-19 and Healthcare System in China: Challenges and Progression for a Sustainable Future," *Globalization and Health* 17, 2021, pp. 14–21.

[112] State Council, "Opinions on Deepening Healthcare Insurance System Reform" ("中共中央國務院關於深化醫療保障制度改革的意見"), http://www.gov.cn/zhengce/2020-03/05/content_5487407.htm (accessed on 15 July 2022).

intend to increase the sustainability of the healthcare insurance system, the fund of the healthcare insurance schemes has suffered a serious deficit during the outbreak of the pandemic.

The data from the National Health Insurance Bureau shows that in the third season in 2021, the basic medical insurance (including maternity insurance) fund income was 625.09 billion *yuan*, of which 626.62 billion *yuan* was spent by the basic medical insurance (including maternity insurance) fund, and the balance was negative (Chart 6.1). Although the overall guarding of the basic medical insurance fund (including the employees' medical insurance fund and the urban and rural residents' medical insurance fund) is still higher than the expenditure, the pressure on the medical insurance fund is unprecedented with the fund's revenue struggling to grow rapidly (Chart 6.2).

The data from the National Health Insurance Bureau also shows that in the third season of 2020, the second season of 2021, the third season of 2021, the second season of 2022, and the third season of 2022, the expenses of the basic medical insurance fund for urban and rural residents exceeded the income, and the balance was negative (Chart 6.3). Although from the pattern of urban and rural residents' basic medical

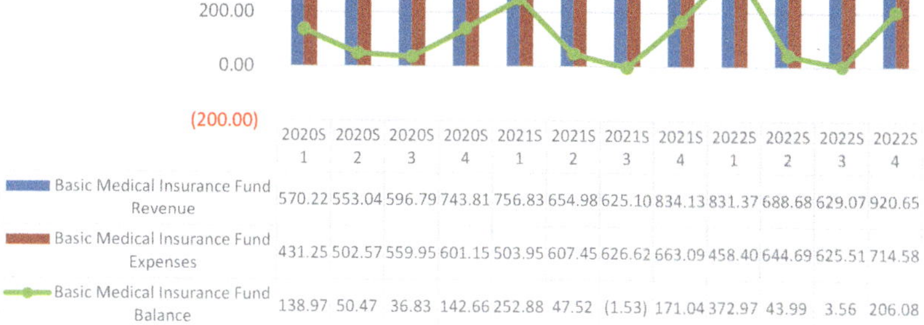

Chart 6.1 Basic medical insurance fund revenue situation (data collected from National Healthcare Security Administration, billion *yuan*)

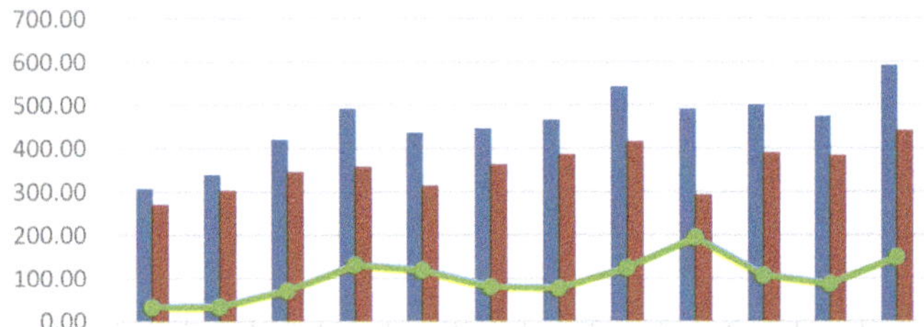

	2020S 1	2020S 2	2020S 3	2020S 4	2021S 1	2021S 2	2021S 3	2021S 4	2022S 1	2022S 2	2022S 3	2022S 4
Employees' Basic Medical Insurance Fund Revenue	308.17	340.51	421.56	492.22	437.68	447.18	467.55	544.39	491.69	501.70	475.71	594.62
Employees' Basic Medical Insurance Fund Expenses	272.85	304.42	347.41	358.72	315.96	364.54	388.10	417.71	295.08	391.85	385.76	443.13
Employees' Basic Medical Insurance Fund Balance	35.32	36.08	74.15	133.51	121.72	82.64	79.45	126.69	196.61	109.84	89.95	151.49

Chart 6.2 Employees' basic medical insurance fund revenue situation (data collected from National Healthcare Security Administration, billion *yuan*)

insurance contributions, it is true that there are individual seasons in a year when income is higher, so from the whole year of 2021 and 2022, there is still a possibility that the fund will return to a positive balance in the current period. But despite this, it still shows that the health insurance fund is faced with severe challenges. Thus, fiscal security continues to be the primary concern for the Chinese social insurance schemes during the Covid-19 pandemic, which will probably result in an insufficient competence of the fragmented social healthcare insurance to inspire citizens' trust toward the capacities in responding to their health needs and interests against healthcare providers (in particular public hospitals).[113]

The other way into this question is to conceive of the rule of law as illustrative of the CCP government's effective venture into the public health emergency management sector. Compared with the measures taken during the SARS outbreak, measures taken in response to the Covid-19 pandemic have achieved significant progress from the standpoint of the rule of law, indicating a further penetration of the rule of law into areas of public health emergency management. In the Chinese government's practices during the SARS outbreak, the laws and regulations were

[113] Mit Ramesh, Xun Wu & Alex Jingwei He, "Health Governance and Healthcare Reforms in China," *Health Policy and Planning* 29(6), 2014, p. 669.

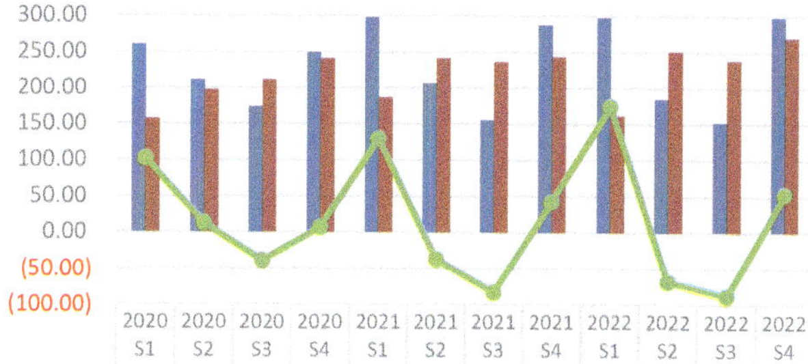

	2020 S1	2020 S2	2020 S3	2020 S4	2021 S1	2021 S2	2021 S3	2021 S4	2022 S1	2022 S2	2022 S3	2022 S4
Residents' Basic Medical Insurance Fund Revenue	262.05	212.54	175.23	251.59	319.15	207.79	157.55	289.73	339.68	186.98	153.36	326.03
Residents' Basic Medical Insurance Fund Expenses	158.40	198.15	212.55	242.43	187.99	242.91	238.52	245.38	163.32	252.84	239.74	271.45
Residents' Basic Medical Insurance Fund Balance	103.65	14.39	(37.32)	9.15	131.16	(35.12)	(80.98)	44.35	176.37	(65.85)	(86.38)	54.59

Chart 6.3 Residents' basic medical insurance fund revenue situation (data collected from National Healthcare Security Administration, billion *yuan*)

not fully observed. As observed by Chenglin Liu, "the PTID had to be re-promulgated by the State Council in order to 'activate' its binding force".[114] This suggests that although the laws and regulations were in effect, they were largely ignored during the SARS outbreak. China's efforts to avoid the reappearance of the SARS crisis and its subsequent effects on economic development and social stability resulted in a number of laws and regulations in the sector of public health emergency management. At a more general level, after President Hu Jintao and Premier Wen Jiabao took power in 2003, the Chinese government was perceived as moving toward "rule by law" rather than a genuine "rule of law".[115] While the narrative of "rule by law" versus "rule of law" continues to be relevant in the Chinese government's responses to the Covid-19 pandemic, the question of the rule of law is more complicated than this. This is because "different degrees of compliance with the rule of law in different domains and contexts of the Chinese state and society" have

[114] Liu, "Regulating SARS in China," 111.

[115] Liebman, "Legal Reform: China's Law-Stability Paradox".

been observed to describe the operation of different areas of the contemporary Chinese legal and judicial systems.[116] This is what appears to be happening during the Covid-19 pandemic. Several observations can be made concerning this.

First, it is crucial to clarify the idea of the rule of law in the context of contemporary Chinese society. Writing of the Chinese judicial and legal systems, Albert Chen suggested the idea of "differential degrees of rule of law in different domains of Chinese society".[117] As observed by Chen, "[i]f the question of the rule of law in China is largely a question of improving compliance with legal norms by both citizens and officials alike—as official discourse seems to suggest—then the problem is relatively simple and the degree to which the rule of law is realized in China is largely an empirical question to be answered by monitoring and measuring the extent of compliance with, or violations of, legal norms".[118] What really matters, as Chen continues, is that the rule of law—as defined by Lon Fuller's eight principles of legality—"is a matter of degree, and it can be realised or complied with in varying degrees in different domains of socioeconomic and sociopolitical life".[119] The idea of the rule of law echoes Fu Hualing's observation and identification of three kinds of practices, i.e., practices based on law, those based on "extra law", and those based on "extra-extra law".[120] Two different degrees of the degrees of the rule of law can be observed in the particular official practices in response to the Covid-19 pandemic.

On the one hand, the Chinese government has been developing laws and regulations in particular after the SARS outbreak. The public health emergency management unites provincial and local governments with functional organs of public health, with myriad laws and regulations at the local level. As noted above, the legal inconsistencies between PCID and the Emergency Law were a reflection of two different logics. The bureaucratic fragmentation of the *tiao-kuai* structure between the public

[116] Chen, Albert, "China's Long March Toward Rule of Law or 'China's Turn Against Law'?" *The Chinese Journal of Comparative Law* 4(1), 2016, p. 30.

[117] *See* ibid.

[118] Ibid., 39–40.

[119] Ibid.

[120] Hualing Fu, "Politicized Challenges, Depoliticized Responses: Political Monitoring in China's Transitions," *University of Hong Kong Faculty of Law Research Paper 2013/014*, 2013.

health organs and the local governments was another factor that resulted in confusion about and denials of the ultimate responsibilities in times of a major pandemic outbreak. The relative status of different government organs of the Chinese fragmented system exacerbated the public health emergency management at the initial stage of the Covid-19 outbreak. The CCDC, a public health institution at the national level, is an entity at the sub-ministry level under the NHC, while the NHC is at the level equivalent to a ministry with the director of the NHC occupying the rank of minister (部長).[121] While the formal status of the minister of the NHC, as a peer of the twenty-five heads of the other commissions and ministries of the central government is parallel to a provincial governor, the public health bureaucracy has not occupied political prominence as the entities governing economy or national security.[122]

Legislative initiatives in this sector also further empowered national regulatory authority. Moreover, the power of the CCDC was still limited. To merge CCDC branches into other government organs at the local level undermined the upward information reporting to the CCDC and exacerbated the orientation of the *kuai* to overshadow *tiao*.[123] Active leadership was needed to ensure that the laws and regulations were able to be flexible and responsive to the public health emergency management to coordinate the hierarchical and functional fragmentation. After the top party leader exercised authority, a sharp contrast could be observed between the early responses of the local governments of Wuhan and Hubei and the later effective design and implementation of the laws and regulations to combat the Covid-19 outbreak. The official practices of the responses to the Covid-19 pandemic demonstrated compliance with laws and regulations under the strong political leadership of the party-state. The practices of complying with laws and regulations could be observed from the large amount of legislations, administrative measures, and judicial interpretations issued after the determination was made by the top political leaders to combat against the Covid-19 pandemic.

[121] Jacques DeLisle & Kui Shen, "China's Response to COVID-19," *Administrative Law Review* 73(1), 2021, p. 34.

[122] Ibid., 35.

[123] Liming Li, Hua Wang, Xiaofeng Liang, et al., "Yiqing Zaoqi, Jibing Yufangkongzhi Tixi Shisheng Yuanyin Hezai?" [疫情早期, 疾病預防控制體系失聲原因何在?] *Intellectual*, http://zhishifenzi.com/depth/depth/8392.html.

On the other hand, the Chinese government also issued secret policies to manage information flow, especially online discussions and activities. The Chinese government's growing ability to manage information and guide online discussions was evident in the processes of dealing with Covid-19 outbreak, but the ability unfolded in the way that took a massive bureaucracy, arms of propaganda team, and digital technology made by private entities. This was what appeared to be happening in Dr. Li Wenliang's death, where, as noted, in case that individual grievances toward the government's disregard of whistleblowers' warning of an unknown disease and the potential of human-to-human transmission were coalescing into a broader protest, the government issued secret government directives, took enormous bureaucracy, specialized technology and armies of people to monitor digital news, gradually removed the name of Li Wenliang, and used fake online commentators to flood websites.[124] The measure was used for the purpose of "trying to defuse the issues and prevent further escalation".[125] This set of official practices, in Fu Hualing's terms and classification, belongs to the practices based on extra law. As defined by Fu, extra law is "defined as an official system in which power is neither directly derived from properly constituted authorities nor subject to independent oversight (judicial or otherwise)".[126] The extra law has some key characteristics, as he continues, including its lack of "deliberation, representation and decision-making that can be regarded as judicial"; these characteristics further give rise to two characteristics that "[i]t has a strong political or policy orientation and the whole system is geared to political expediency or convenience".[127] As put by Fu, the Chinese media governance is "essentially a lawless business" with traditional media as strictly controlled by licensing requirements, strong demands on professional participation, and state authority with party

[124] Raymond Zhong, Paul Mozur & Aaron Krolik, "Leaked Documents Show How China's Army of Paid Internet Trolls Helped Censor the Coronavirus," *ProPublica & New York Times*, https://www.propublica.org/article/leaked-documents-show-how-chinas-army-of-paid-internet-trolls-helped-censor-the-coronavirus.

[125] Fu, "Politicized Challenges, Depoliticized Responses," p. 25.

[126] Ibid., 27.

[127] Hualing Fu, "The Varieties of Law," https://lawprofessors.typepad.com/china_law_prof_blog/2011/06/fu-hualing-on-the-varieties-of-law.html.

discipline.[128] With a combination of the formal conventions and self-disciplinary commitments, government directives as a kind of "extra law" constituted a set of regulatory measures that embodied "the increasingly intricate envelope for permitted speech".[129] In this sense, while freedom of speech and particular forms of communication are allowed, they are only permitted within the specific framework defined by the party-state through the creation of the "extra-law" measures.

Second, the preceding observation regarding the rule of law invites us to revisit the view that the Chinese measures to fight against the Covid-19 pandemic were simply a reinforcement of the paternalist campaign mode of crisis governance. For some commentators, the "*paternalist campaign-style mode of crisis governance* has not diminished in the current response to Covid-19, but has in fact strengthened".[130] The perception of the Chinese party-state's power as a "campaign-style mode of crisis governance", however, neglects some nuances of the improvement of different public health emergency management capacities, which has enabled the party-state to play a more assertive role—due to the effective combination of the economic, military, and ideological power—than that during the patriotic hygiene campaign and the SARS outbreak. As noted above, in paternalist patriotic campaigns in the 1950s, while the party-state had despotic power it had limited infrastructural power, i.e., the institutional capacity to penetrate and coordinate actors of the communities.[131]

After the SARS outbreak, there were more laws and regulations and more effective capacity building for public health emergency management, which allowed the party-state to penetrate and coordinate public health emergency management activities. The Chinese government also began to strengthen social welfare. The political will and fiscal capacity have enabled the Chinese government to expand the scope of universal basic health care. In 2002, various forms of medical insurance were introduced in urban China, with the basic medical insurance system for urban workers increasing from 15.1 million in 1998 to 200.5 million in

[128] *See* Creemers, "The Privilege of Speech and New Media".

[129] Fu, "Politicized Challenges, Depoliticized Responses," p. 27.

[130] Alex Jingwei He, Yuda Shi & Hongdou Liu, "Crisis Governance, Chinese Style: Distinctive Features of China's Response to the Covid-19 Pandemic," *Policy Design and Practice* 3(3), 2020.

[131] In the term of Michael Mann, the power of the state has two important aspects of power, i.e., despotic power and infrastructural power.

2008.[132] On April 6, 2009, the Chinese government issued the Guideline of Healthcare Reform, pledging to expand basic health insurance coverage to 90% of all citizens by 2011 and to realize the provision of "safe, effective, convenient and affordable" basic healthcare services to all citizens by 2020.[133]

During the Covid-19 outbreak, unlike during the SARS outbreak, patients' treatment and medical expenses are fully covered by the Social Medical Security Fund and public finances. The expansion of medical staff and resources after the SARS outbreak has also made it possible to use designated hospitals to consolidate patients, treatment, and medical resources.[134]

Apart from the Emergency Management Law enacted in 2007, there were five types of emergency events regulated by law, including wars, natural disasters, accidents and disasters, public health events, and social security events. In April 2018, in accordance with the "Plan for Deepening Party and State Institutional Reform" of the Third Plenary Session of the 19th Party Central Committee, the Department of Emergency Management was officially established.[135] The Ministry integrates 13 responsibilities of 11 departments and the responsibilities of 5 national command and coordination agencies. Thus, the infrastructural power of the party-state has been gradually developed, with a more institutionalized form of public health emergency management and social actors passing through the command structure of the party-state. While the despotic power is still strong during the Covid-19 outbreak, the infrastructural power of the party-state is more advanced than during the patriotic hygiene campaign.

In addition, digital technology has become an important element in improving the party-state's ability to penetrate further into the public health emergency management sector. With the digital technology of

[132] Shaoguang Wang, "China's Double Movement in Health Care," *Socialist Register* 46, 2010, p. 264.

[133] Ibid., 266.

[134] Fujun Peng, Lei Tu, Yongshi Yang, et al., "Management and Treatment of COVID-19: The Chinese Experience," *Canadian Journal of Cardiology* 36(6), 2020, p. 917.

[135] Ministry of Emergency Management: Emergency management system with Chinese characteristics has been basically formed [應急管理部: 中國特色應急管理體制基本形成], https://www.gov.cn/xinwen/2022-08/31/content_5707517.htm.

surveillance and tracking in operation, more sensitive public health emergency management was made possible by the health QR code system. Suspected patients could be accurately identified and isolated to a specific area without placing the entire county or city in a state of emergency. The widespread use of surveillance for disease prevention and control during the Covid-19 pandemic reinforces the concern that both laws and cyber norms can provide a basis for guiding people's actions. China used surveillance of individuals' location histories to create infection risk scoring systems, and also required citizens to score and show "green" to enter public places, workplaces, and so on.[136] Digital contact tracing was designed as a public health tool, but it was also used as a permit to return to work in China. This technology not only allowed for a less visible and more automatic means of control and social surveillance to isolate and report citizens' behavior through digital applications for broader surveillance purposes. While the creation of digital contact tracing was authorized by law, the modes of digital contact tracing technology also played a role in reinventing the law.[137] From this point of view, unlike in the years before the SARS outbreak, when the party-state primarily withdrew from socioeconomic management, the party-state now has the capacity to penetrate the field of public health emergency management in a regularized manner.

Third, to the extent that law and the rule of law have penetrated more deeply into the domain of public health emergency management than they did after the SARS outbreak, the upgrading of the rule of law requires a reconsideration of the form of legitimation through legality throughout public health emergency management. As explained earlier, the form of legitimation under the Maoist mobilization-based patriotic hygiene movement could be thought to "[t]o accord with the mass line, leaders in the formulation of policies must go among the masses, listen to their views, systematize them, and take the results back to the masses".[138] During the SARS outbreak, it turned out that while the Maoist mobilization-based management was effective in mobilizing

136 Glenn Cohen, Lawrence O. Gostin & Daniel J. Weitzner, "Digital Smartphone Tracking for COVID-19: Public Health and Civil Liberties in Tension," *Jama* 323(23), 2020, p. 2371.

137 Lydia Khalil, "Digital Authoritarianism, China and Covid," https://www.lowyinstitute.org/publications/digital-authoritarianism-china-and-covid.

138 Tsou, "Interpreting the Revolution in China," pp. 216–7.

resources to curb the spread of the disease without professional guidance and institutionalization, the SARS outbreak revealed not only institutional weaknesses of the public health emergency management, but even the whole political system. As David Fidler once commented, "China still looms large in any future confrontation with SARS, raising concerns about China's attitude should the virus and disease return. As a group of public health experts observed, '[m]any of the solutions to solve the multifaceted puzzle of SARS and to prevent future epidemics must come from China'". China suppressing the debate on political reform after the SARS outbreak creates worries and fears about whether China will provide transparent and timely responses to the outbreak of novel diseases. After the SARS outbreak, the party-state revised the outdated legislations of information reporting.

During the Covid-19 pandemic, moreover, the shift to the rule of law was a reflection of the Chinese government's legitimation demand for the rule of law. At a general level, the rule of law is demanded by the party-state as the direction of its mode of governance. As the "study guide" issued in 2017 on Xi's 19th Party Congress speech said, "only by governing the country according to law", the document continues, "can we liberate and strengthen the productive energies of society, promote social justice, maintain social harmony and stability, and sustain the long-term peace and viability of both the Party and the country at large".[139] In addition, during a novel infectious disease emergency, the rule of law is critical to increasing the predictability, transparency, and reliability of government action, which helps to reduce citizen panic and restore confidence in the socioeconomic order. Unlike the crisis governance of ordinary natural disasters, infectious diseases have some unique characteristics. First, while the physical damage caused by natural disasters such as hurricanes and earthquakes may be limited to their original impact areas, outbreaks of infectious diseases can spread far beyond the epicenter, along with the self-replication of infected pathogens.[140] The government faces significant challenges in responding to outbreaks in multiple locations simultaneously. Second, unlike natural diseases whose causes

[139] People's Daily Online, "Why Should We Adhere to the Comprehensive Rule of Law?" [為什麼要堅持全面依法治國], http://cpc.people.com.cn/n1/2017/1130/c415067-29677669.html.

[140] *See* Huang, *Governing Health in Contemporary China*.

are secondary to rescue and relief efforts, rapid and accurate identification of the etiology of an unknown disease and a novel and emerging pathogen is critical to an effective response. However, the emergence of an unknown disease is often associated with diagnostic delays and misdiagnosis. Uncertainty is also inherent in dealing with the emergence of a novel disease. "We respond to the likelihood of death in the event the disease is contracted, rather than the compound probability of contracting the disease and succumbing to its effects".[141] The uncertainty associated with the response to the disease often generates panic, the level of which may be disproportionate to the mortality caused by the disease. Third, unlike a natural disaster, which can typically generate increased sympathy and interaction, an unknown disease is often associated with isolation, social distancing, widespread fear, and restrictions on commerce and international trade. In 2005, a flock of chickens in Colombia was infected with avian influenza. After Colombia reported the outbreak to the WHO, five neighboring countries banned poultry from Colombia. In this sense, a government that discovers the emergence of novel infectious diseases often faces a dilemma between disclosing the potential outbreak and the negative socioeconomic consequences of disclosure. Thus, given the unique characteristics of a novel disease outbreak, the rule of law is critical to enhancing the reliability of government actions, averting public panic, and restoring confidence in the socioeconomic order.

As the three illustrative examples illustrated in this chapter attest, the Chinese public health emergency management system has been subject to changes driven by an increasing emphasis on effective prevention and control of public health emergencies. As noted by Bourdieu when writing of "the force of law",

> In Bourdieu's conception a social field is the site of struggle, of competition for control. (Indeed, the field defines what is to be controlled: it locates the issues about which dispute is socially meaningful, and thus those concerning which a victory is desirable).[142]

[141] Jessica Stern, "Dreaded Risks and the Control of Biological Weapons," *International Security* 27(3) Winter 2002/03, p. 105.

[142] Pierre Bourdieu, "The Force of Law: Toward a Sociology of the Juridical Field," *The Hastings Law Journal* 38, 1986, p. 808.

After the SARS outbreak, the legal and institutional sides of Chinese public health emergency management have begun to take shape as a field of practice. As the public health emergency management becomes a field with multiple sites of intersection between public health and emergency management, it has been built on different main pillars of the two sites, which shows conflicts in their responses to the Covid-19 pandemic at the initial stage. This suggests that the current field of Chinese public health emergency management is one in which the struggle over its development and future direction continues to be a pressing issue. By excavating some of the legacies of the patriotic hygiene campaigns of the 1950s, one of the contributions of this chapter is to highlight the dynamism and responsiveness envisioned at their inception. This is not only to analyze how the laws and institutional arrangements of public health emergency management differ from those that emerged in the 1950s, but also to contrast them with the legacy of the campaigns in today's development and reform of China's public health system.

CHAPTER 7

Bringing Trust to Physician–Patient Relationship

7.1 Reconfiguring Physician Obligations

To rebuild trust between physicians and patients, it must open the door to the ethics of responsibility in decision-making to ensure that informed consent, and patient autonomy more broadly, cannot be divorced from the establishment of caring relationships and the obligations of providing care to patients. The value of informed consent must be understood not only as the protection of personal autonomy, but also as the assurance that patients trust physicians. To explain the ethical account of trust and obligation, this chapter draws on theories of the ethics of care and offers suggestions for improving the trusting relationship between physicians and patients.

The ethical discussion of medical ethics emphasizes the relationship between people as equal subjects. It has four components that are crucial to improving the trust relationship between physicians and patients in contemporary China. The first component of the ethics of care is attention or engagement. Attention must be given to the caregiver. In the absence of the cared-for, reflection is crucial for caregivers to reflect on their role as role models. The second component of the ethics of care is dialogue. Caregivers must give attention, or at least momentary attention, to the cared-for, while the cared-for must receive attention. In genuine dialogue, attention is given not only to intellectual objects but also to the

L. Jia, *Obligation*, IPP Studies in the Frontiers of China's Public Policy,
https://doi.org/10.1007/978-981-99-6437-6_7

participants. Dialogue can also have multiple episodes. As noted by Nel Noddings,

> True dialogue ... is open-ended. The participants do not know at the outset what the conclusions will be. Both speak; both listen. Dialogue is not just conversation. There must be a topic, but the topic may shift, and either party in a dialogue may divert attention from the original topic to one more crucial, or less sensitive, or more fundamental.[1]

Dialogue allows information to be shared in a safe environment and encourages reflection and thought. Dialogue also provides a way of acknowledging the presence of the other and responding to the needs of the other.

The third component is practice, in the sense that the capacity for interpersonal attention needs to be developed through engagement in caring activities, such as working in small groups, community service, and so on.[2] The fourth component is confirmation. According to Noddings, confirmation "requires a relation. Carers have to understand their cared-fors well enough to know what it is they are trying to accomplish".[3] This suggests that affirmation is not something that can be given as a ritual act; rather, it must be offered on the basis that a genuine dialogue has established a relationship that allows the parties to acknowledge what they really need or want.[4]

What are the implications of the ethics of care for understanding physician–patient relationships of trust? First, the restoration of trusting relationships between doctors and patients requires the fulfillment of the ethics of responsibility. The decline of trust between physicians and patients is part of the broader and deeper social crisis in which the core of obligation, that is, the bond or common glue between one another, has been weakened.[5] Trustworthiness requires the mutual commitment of each other, so it is the ethics of responsibility that forms the moral

[1] Ibid.

[2] Ibid., 19.

[3] Ibid., 21.

[4] Ibid.

[5] Alfred Tauber, "In Search of Medicine's Moral Glue," *American Journal of Bioethics* 6(1), 2006, p. 41.

foundation of the trusting relationship.[6] In the medical context, patients are subject to multiple sources of vulnerability, such as poor economic conditions, psychological vulnerability of illness, and the condition of the illness, the patient's trust arises from the physician's responsiveness to the illness.[7] However, physicians are not only responsive to the needs of patients. Physicians work within a set of professional responsibilities that require them to be responsive to the institutions in which they work.[8] Physicians thus have to be subject to many different kinds of obligations. Although the different kinds of obligations may conflict with one another, no matter what kind of decisions physicians ultimately make their actions "follow from judgments and options governed by an array of considerations governed by the patient's best interests at various levels".[9] Patient trust in physicians emerges when patients realize that physicians focus on care taking of patients and other competing matters are subordinated.[10] This requires a process ethics. As put by Tauber, "[t]his 'process' ethics, dynamic and dialectical, requires a moral compass. Physicians are constantly making value judgments ranging from interpretations of data, to choosing a clinical strategy, to forming relationships with patients and hospital personnel".[11]

Second, the ethics of care demands a number of responsibilities for physicians and patients to act in ways that enhance their trusting relationship. For example, it requires physicians to listen, respond emotionally, and communicate with patients and their family members. Physicians should use their emotions, cognitions, personalities, and values therapeutically.[12] In addition, physicians are encouraged to engage in critical self-reflection about the ethical issues in medical practice, including the barriers that may impede the delivery of care. For example, the healthcare financing system can be a major barrier that prevents physicians in many

[6] Ibid., 42.

[7] Ibid.

[8] Ibid.; *see* also Ezekiel Emanuel & Linda L. Emanuel, "What Is Accountability in Health Care?," *Annals of Internal Medicine* 124(2), 1996.

[9] Ibid.

[10] Ibid.

[11] Ibid.

[12] Arthur Kleinman, "Caregiving: Its Role in Medicine and Society in America and China," *Ageing International* 35, 2010, p. 104.

countries from spending more time communicating with patients. This ethical responsibility to provide care not only requires physicians to identify the problems and barriers in medical practice, but also to resist and correct them.[13] It is also required to redefine the concept of sickness and disease as a kind of social suffering of human beings.[14] To shift the focus of physicians' attention from health and medicine to a large-scale process of economic, political, and cultural changes in human beings that have contributed not only to the emergence of social and mental health problems but also to the deterioration of healthcare financing situations. As a result, physicians will be aware of the importance of health inequalities and poverty among populations.[15] When physicians critically reflect on the ethical issues of social and health policy, they would realize that their reflections affect not only the disease conditions of individual patients, but also the health conditions, poverty, and health disparities of populations.

Third, restoring the relationship of trust may give rise to a number of duties, including the duty of loyalty and the duty of care. The specification of the duty of care varies from relationship to relationship, depending on the nature of the power exercised by the stronger party and how the interests of the weaker party can be defined. But this simple statement belies the difficulty of specifying the scope of the duties. For example, in the case of McInerney vs. MacDonald, the patient demanded a copy of her medical records. The physician released only the medical record she had prepared, while refusing to release records prepared by other physicians. The patient went to court to get a copy of the records. Justice La Forest J. wrote that the physician–patient relationship was fiduciary because of the "trust and confidence" placed in the physician when the intimate details of the patient's life were shared with the physician. This relationship of trust and confidence gave rise to the "[f]iduciary duty to provide access to medical records ... Information about oneself revealed to a doctor acting in a professional capacity remains in a fundamental sense, one's own. The doctor's position is one of trust and confidence. The information conveyed is held in a fashion somewhat akin to a trust ... The confiding of the information to the physician for medical purposes

[13] Ibid., 105.

[14] Arthur Kleinman, Veena Das, and Margaret Lock, eds., *Social Suffering*, Berkeley: University of California Press, 1997.

[15] Kleinman, "Caregiving," p. 106.

gives rise to an expectation that the patient's interest in and control the information will continue".[16] In this case, Justice La Forest regarded the patient's access to her medical records as "prima facie the patient's best interests" and this right was derived from the physician's duty to act with loyalty and good faith as a fiduciary.

Incorporating fiduciary duties into Chinese medical law would make the ethical duties of informed consent independent obligations. For example, in Chinese medical practice, physicians may receive red bags from medical device manufacturers or their agents. Physicians and medical device manufacturers may then collude to induce patients to purchase and use the latter's products during the treatment process. This problem is very common in China, as evidenced by the fact that many patients have opted for stents instead of bypass surgery. The international ratio of stents to bypass surgery is 7:1 to 8:1, but in China this ratio is as high as 12:1. Moreover, while it is generally believed that few patients need more than 3 cardiac stents, many patients in China have as many as 10 cardiac stents.[17] When this kind of case is brought to court, a judge may apply the fiduciary duties to produce the liabilities for violating the ethical duties of informed consent independent of personal injuries. The fiduciaries take advantage of the fiduciary status to impose extra charges on the beneficiaries. In the case of imposing undue influences and seeking personal economic gains, when it is dealt in accordance with the legal consequences of violating fiduciary duties, the trustee's benefits should be repaid and illegal benefits should eventually be returned to patients. When the violation of the duties of informed consent is accompanied by such an independent liability induced by the fiduciary duties physicians and hospitals will be incentivized to reduce the purchase and use of the unnecessary yet costly medical products, while paying more attention to the actual health needs of patients.

In this sense, an effective implementation of the doctrine of informed consent depends on the formation of a trusting relationship between physicians and patients, while a genuine and sincere communication

[16] McInerney v. MacDonald, 1992 CanLII 57 (SCC), [1992] 2 SCR 138.

[17] Global Times, "Doctors induce patients to place heart stents" [醫生誘導患者放置心臟支架: 國外用 3 個國內用 10 個], https://china.huanqiu.com/article/9CaKrnK1Flk.

between physicians and patients also contributes to the trusting relationship between physicians and patients. In other words, the formation of a trusting relationship and the implementation of the doctrine of informed consent may constitute a virtuous circle.

7.2 Reconfiguring Patient Obligations

Shifting the focus of medical practice in contemporary China from administrative regulation and marketization to the responsibility of caring also requires the fulfillment of patients' obligations. The essence of caring is a kind of reciprocity. Reciprocity is different from financial exchange and close to the exchange of gifts between people. In return for the things done by caregivers, the person being cared-for also needs to share his or her experiences and stories.[18] From this point of view, the physician has to take on obligations toward the patient; and in doing so, the physician and the patient are characterized as being responsible for each other.

Here it is crucial to focus on the bond or tie that lies at the core of obligation. By reference to Birks's account of Roman Law that "[a]n obligation is a rope … by which we are tied", Scott Veitch points out that a person's legal obligation has "its antecedents in the fact that he was literally 'bound to' do it".[19] Solidarity, in the form of joint liability, is the bonding force that ties people together. In Roman Law,

> *obligation in solidum* defines the status of *joint liability* for a financial debt … To be in solidarity means that a man is good for his debts and stands up to his obligations to others even when he has not benefited from them directly. To be the cosignatory of a loan means that one is liable for the reversals of fortune of another; that one's own economic well-being is no longer completely in one's own hands.[20]

What is emphasized here is not only how creditors and debtors create bonds between them, but the notion of joint liability plays the role of tying people together. In other words, it is the existence of joint liability

[18] Arthur Kleinman, "Caregiving as Moral Experience," *The Lancet* 380(9853), 2012, p. 1551.

[19] Ibid., 425.

[20] Emphasis added, Veitch, *Obligations*, p. 102.

that makes the collective greater than the sum of individual parts of the collective.

As noted above, Nie is correct in pointing out that informed consent contributes to promoting the bond of mutual trust between physicians and patients, but he does not specify how to establish the bond of trust between physicians and patients. The conventional understanding of informed consent only asserts that competent patients should be allowed to have information, make decisions for themselves regarding the course of their medical interventions, whereas physicians should communicate effectively with patients and/or their family members. Little has been said about what kind of decisions should be made by patients, as well as whether patients should take responsibilities for making decisions.

Recent ethical discussions of patient responsibility may help to clarify how to reconfigure the patient obligations correlative to the right to informed consent to restore the bond of trust between physicians and patients in contemporary China. Draper and Sorell argue that, given that patients usually need to bear the consequences of their decisions, physicians may rescue them from the consequences of their decisions. Although patients are vulnerable, their vulnerability does not confer inability to make bad health outcomes. Nor does their autonomy insulate them from their responsibility for the outcomes of their decisions. Draper and Sorell's idea of patient responsibility points to an ideal type of a genuine partnership between physicians and patients in medical treatment, which demands a "joint responsibility for the outcomes, including cases where things go badly wholly as a result of these decisions, and the patient turns out to be harmed or disappointed".[21] In this sense, Draper and Sorell's article supplements Nie's argument on the point the performance of both physician and patient obligations helps to form the bond between them.

As physicians have obligations to be sensitive to patients, such as to truthfully inform patients or their family members of the patients' conditions without incurring adverse impacts on patients, patients also have obligations to attend to physicians, for instance, to actively communicate with physicians, engaging themselves in decision-making and taking liability for the outcomes of decisions. By taking the form of normative specification, it specifies particular types of obligations that citizens

[21] Heather Draper & Tom Sorell, "Patients' Responsibilities in Medical Ethics," *Bioethics* 16(4), 2002, pp. 339–40.

as obligation bearers should have. Apart from specifying the state's obligations, the Basic Health Law demands individual obligations, as citizens are also important bearers of obligations. The Basic Health Law engages with what is called here the civic sense of individual obligation. It has three key features related to the theme discussed in this book.

First, by taking the form of normative specification, it specifies the particular types of obligations citizens as obligation bearers should have. Pursuant to Art 57,[22] citizens should not be merely passive recipients of health care; rather, they have obligations to respect medical professionals. The obligations to respect medical professionals flow from a general obligation for everyone to respect others.[23] The general obligation to respect others is owed to everyone, not just physicians or nurses. Anyone who swears at or punches others without provocation is doing something disrespectful, something wrong. The obligation to respect physicians is particularly important in that it is even more disrespectful to punch those who they are trying to help.

Second, the Basic Health Law also stipulates self-binding obligations that citizens should have to promote their own health. This is specified by the specification of the Basic Health Law. Art 69(1) provides that, "Citizens are the primary obligation bearers for their own health". They are obligated "to establish and to practice good ideas of health management so as to be responsible for their own health, take the initiative to acquire health knowledge, improve health literacy, and strengthen health management ..." Art 69(2) further specifies that, "Citizens should respect the health rights and interests of others, and shall not damage the health rights of others and the public health interests". Citizens are required to reflect on their lifestyle, to take measures that promote their health and prevent illness, and to adopt preventative measures suggested by their physicians. This series of obligations in this sense can be characterized as self-binding.

Third, the self-binding obligations have an other-regarding dimension as they are related to the solidarity (the bond) between citizens—which suggests that they owe obligations to other citizens. This type of patient obligation is grounded on obligations as citizens, regarding how to treat

[22] Art 57 specifies that "the whole society should care and respect medical and health professionals, maintain a good and safe order of medical and health service, and jointly build a harmonious physician-patient relationship".

[23] Draper & Sorell, "Patients' Responsibilities in Medical Ethics," p. 340.

other citizens who are bound together by the healthcare insurance system with finite public resources.[24] For instance, if one is advised by his doctor to drink or smoke less, and he disregards this advice, when his health deteriorates, leading to the consequence that costly treatment and enormous health resources must be invested to rescue him, he may fail to discharge the obligations to preserve his health. In this sense, the observance of obligations derivable from the idea of patients as citizens—say, respecting physicians, listening to their advice of taking preventive measures, and living a healthy lifestyle—posits a form of solidarity (in terms of joint liability) between citizens in the healthcare context, which constitutes an extension of the sphere of autonomy of patients and the solidarity between physicians and patients to encompass all citizens. This form of solidarity between citizens is also the ground of the legal obligations to be assumed by the state (as specified by the objective of the healthcare reform) to provide citizens a basic healthcare service.

[24] For the idea of linking patients' obligations with the interests of other patients, *see* Martyn Evans, "Do Patients have Duties," *Journal of Medical Ethics* 33(12), 2007.

Conclusion

This book has attempted to chart the historical shifts in the particular form of the physician–patient relationship and the nature of physician–patient obligations in the context of China's healthcare reforms. These shifts are the result of policy choices made by the state. Against the historical backdrop of the collective economy in rural China, China once developed and implemented the barefoot doctor program as an effective way of providing healthcare and created a corresponding form of physician–patient relationship with a strong bond of mutual trust. As the literature cited in this book attests, the changing nature of physician–patient obligations has been subject to many factors, i.e., political control, close-knit communities, decommodification of healthcare, etc. In the two subsequent rounds of healthcare reform, some of the economic factors—particularly the commodification and marketization of healthcare—have deeply shaped the expectations and practices of physicians and patients, and they have also altered the once-robust understanding of physician and patient obligations.

Moreover, in the context of the marketization of healthcare, the physician–patient relationship was caught in a vicious circle of worsening mistrust. Despite the implementation of the right to informed consent and other legal mechanisms in the field of healthcare, the physician–patient bond threatened to collapse. Law and legal institutions during this period facilitated, rather than prevented, the disconnection of medical practice from ethical obligation. Although the introduction of

L. Jia, *Obligation*, IPP Studies in the Frontiers of China's Public Policy,
https://doi.org/10.1007/978-981-99-6437-6

the public contract and the public hospital reform tended to reaffirm the decommodification of healthcare and the establishment of the bond of citizenship, which was presumably to improve physician–patient relations, the two different approaches to the current round of healthcare reform suggested the existence of a political struggle and contestation over the approaches to managing the healthcare reform. The contestation over the future direction of health reform continues to be a live and debated issue. By excavating some of the origins of the barefoot doctors' sense of ethical obligation, this book has to recall the bond of trust between physicians and patients at that time. By identifying and discussing examples of recent rounds of healthcare reform, such as the legal implementation of the notion of informed consent, the right to health, public contracting, public hospital reform, etc., this book has not only enabled an analysis of how the bond of trust between physicians and patients, and between the state and the citizen, has changed over time, but has also highlighted the vulnerability of patients (and citizens in general) when the bonds of trust threaten to collapse.

To better understand the physician–patient relationship and the citizen–state relationship, this book has also discussed people's trust in the public health emergency management system. As of the writing of this book, the Covid-19 pandemic has gripped the nations of the world for nearly three years. It observes that while the law has been used by the Chinese government as a legitimizing mode of public health emergency management, the extra-legal practices continue to operate during Covid-19. While suspicions about China's propensity for governance by law remain, China's public health emergency management system has been subject to change, driven by an increasing emphasis on transparency. The Notice of Consultation for the revision of the PTID was issued in October 2020.[1] One important proposal is to expand the scope of government agencies to include the county CDC to promptly issue early warnings of infectious diseases, thereby eliminating its inconsistencies with the Emergency Response Law. In this sense, while the features of the emergency disciplinary state have far-reaching implications for China's subsequent public health emergency management, to the extent that the

[1] NHC, "National Health Commission Notice of Public Consultation on Revising the Law of the People's Republic of China on the Prevention and Control of Infectious Diseases," 2 October 2020, http://www.nhc.gov.cn/wjw/yjzj/202010/330ecbd72c3940408c3e5a49e8651343.shtm.

role of law has gradually improved in the public health emergency scheme during SARS and Covid-19 pandemic, China's public health emergency management scheme has shown an increased level of transparency.

After explaining that people's trust in public hospitals (and the health-care system in general) may be declining due to the significant restrictions on healthcare funding during the Covid-19 pandemic, this book has returned to the physician–patient relationship in China. The initiation of the current round of healthcare reform across China, although it intends to provide healthcare as a public good, the concrete healthcare policies also reveal an erosion of the dual logic of bureaucratic control and market competitiveness. From this point of view, as China scales up the pilot initiative of systemic health reform, it must not only improve the purchasing capacity of the healthcare insurance funds, but also expand the roles and functions of the healthcare insurance funds to include the obligations of increasing their responsiveness to the health needs of patients. To this end, in addition to improving competition between healthcare insurance schemes to provide better conditions of healthcare services to their members, strengthening the performance of the other-regarding obligation or the bond with others can be linked to two aspects of concrete legal and policy proposals. On the one hand, the recent opinions of the State Council highlight its emphasis on the regulatory obligations and roles of healthcare insurance systems in responding to the health needs of citizens. If the State Council's opinions can be effectively implemented through concrete social and health policies as planned, citizens' trust in health insurance systems can be improved; otherwise, to the extent that citizens have limited power to express their health needs and interests, their vulnerability to healthcare providers will be aggravated and their sense of financial anxiety in case of illness may not be eliminated.

On the other hand, citizens should not be passive recipients of health-care; rather, they have an obligation to respect medical professionals and to conserve the state's healthcare resources. The Basic Health Law has addressed what might be called the civic sense of individual obligation. The fulfillment of the obligations derived from the idea of patients as citizens contributes to the formation and maintenance of solidarity among citizens. Since the fulfillment of these obligations by citizens also contributes to saving the state's healthcare resources, the bond between citizens and healthcare insurance companies will be strengthened.

Bibliography

21st Century Business Herald, "China's CDC System 'Epidemic' Change: Upgrading, Integration, Synergy, Sinking" [中國疾控體系"疫"變：升格、整合、協同、下沉], https://m.21jingji.com/article/20210512/846b0b8a1047ae55bb76280fe9a019bb.html.

Baier, Annette, "Trust and Antitrust," *Ethics* 96(2), 1986.

———, *Moral Prejudices: Essays on Ethics*, Cambridge: Harvard University Press, 1994.

Barthes, Roland, *The Semiotic Challenge*, Berkeley, CA: University of California Press, 1994.

BBC News, "The History of the NHS in Charts," https://www.bbc.co.uk/news/health-44560590.

———, "The NHS: 'One of the greatest achievements in history'," http://news.bbc.co.uk/2/hi/events/nhs_at_50/special_report/123511.stm.

Beaglehole, Robert and Ruth Bonita, "Public Health Themes: Historical and Contemporary," *Public Health at the Crossroads: Achievements and Prospects*, Cambridge: Cambridge University Press, 1997.

Benjamin, Liebman, "Malpractice Mobs: Medical Dispute Resolution in China," *Columbia Law Review* 113(1), 2013.

Bevan, Aneurin, *In Place of Fear*, Read Books Ltd, 2011.

Bok, Sissela, *Secrets: On the Ethics of Concealment and Revelation*, New York: Pantheon Books, 1982.

Bossons, Matthew, "Pregnant Woman's Suicide Spurs Heated Debate in China," https://www.thatsmags.com/china/post/20539/pregnant-woman-s-suicide-spurs-heated-debated-in-china.

L. Jia, *Obligation*, IPP Studies in the Frontiers of China's Public Policy, https://doi.org/10.1007/978-981-99-6437-6

Bouey, Jennifer, "China's Health System Reform and Global Health Strategy in the Context of COVID-19," *Rand*, 2020.

Bourdieu, Pierre, "The Force of Law: Toward a Sociology of the Juridical Field," *The Hastings Law Journal* 38, 1986.

Brazier, Margaret, "Do No Harm-Do Patients Have Responsibilities Too?," *Cambridge Law Journal* 65, 2005.

Caixin, "31 Provinces of China Initiated Level-One Response to Public Health Emergency" [中國內地31省份全部啓動突發公共衛生事件一級回應], http://china.caixin.com/2020-01-29/101509411.html.

Cao, Jingchun, "Protecting the Right to Privacy in China," *Victoria University of Wellington Law Review* 36, 2005.

Cao, Yongfu Yunling Wang and Linjuan Zheng, "Towards a Confucian Approach to Health Care Allocation in China: A Dynamic Geography," in Julia Tao, ed., *China: Bioethics, Trust, and the Challenge of the Market*, 2008.

Central Commission for Discipline Inspection of the Communist Party of China, "The Central Committee of the Communist Party of China: To Carry Out Large-Scale Nucleic Acid and Antibody Testing," http://www.ccdi.gov.cn/toutiao/202004/t20200424_216055.html.

Central Intelligence Agency, "SARS: Lesson from the First Epidemic of the 21st Century: A Collaborative Analysis with Outside Experts".

Cha, Cheris Shun-Ching, "Mistrust of Physicians in China, Society, Institution and Interaction as Root Causes," *Developing World Bioethics* 18(1), 2018.

Chen, Albert, "China's Long March Toward Rule of Law' or 'China's Turn Against Law'?," *The Chinese Journal of Comparative Law* 4(1), 2016.

Chen, C.C., *Medicine in Rural China: A Personal Account*, Berkeley, Los Angeles, London: University of California Press.

Chen, Mengji, Shan Xu, Lewis Husain and Gauden Galea, "Digital Health Interventions for Covid-19 in China: A Retrospective Analysis," *Intelligent Medicine* 1(1), 2021.

Chen, Zhuo, "COVID-19 and the Case for Empowering China's CDC," *Sixth Tone*, March 28, 2020.

Cheng, Xiao, "On the Obligations of Medical Practitioners in Civil Disputes over Medical Damages [論醫療損害民事糾紛中醫療者的義務]," *Modern Drug Applications in China* 4 [中國現代藥物應用], 2008.

Chenglin, Liu, "Regulating SARS in China: Law as an Antidote?," *Washington University Law Review* 4(1), 2005.

China Health Yearbook [中國衛生統計年鑒], Beijing: Remin Weisheng Press, 1983.

CNR News, "Behind the 17,000 *yuan* Per Capita Medical Cost of Covid-19 Patients: A People-Centered Health Insurance System" [新冠肺炎患者人均醫療費用1.7萬元背後: 以人民為中心的醫保制度], http://news.cnr.cn/native/gd/20200331/t20200331_525036902.shtml.

Coase, Ronald, *The Firm, the Market and the Law*, Chicago: University of Chicago Press, 1988.

Cohen, Glenn, Lawrence O. Gostin and Daniel J. Weitzner, "Digital Smartphone Tracking for COVID-19: Public Health and Civil Liberties in Tension," *Jama* 323(23), 2020.

Cong, Yali, "Doctor-Family-Patient Relationship: The Chinese Paradigm of Informed Consent," *The Journal of Medicine and Philosophy* 29(2), 2004.

Craig, Paul, *Administrative Law*, London: Sweet & Maxwell, 2021.

Creemers, Rogier, "The Privilege of Speech and New Media: Conceptualizing China's Communications Law in the Internet Age," in Jacques DeLisle, Avery Goldstein and Guobin Yang, eds., *Internet, Social Media and a Changing China*, Pennsylvania: University of Pennsylvania Press, 2016.

———, "Cyber China: Upgrading Propaganda, Public Opinion Work and Social Management for the Twenty-First Century," *Journal of Contemporary China* 26, 2017.

Daniels, Norman, *Just Health Care*, Cambridge: Cambridge University Press, 1985.

De Villiers, Bertus, "Directive Principles of State Policy and Fundamental Rights: The Indian Experience," *South African Journal on Human Rights* 8(1), 1992.

DeLisle, Jacques and Kui Shen, "China's Response to COVID-19," *Administrative Law Review* 73(1), 2021, p. 35.

Delanda, Manuel, *War in the Age of Intelligent Machines*, New York: Swerwe Editions, 1991.

Ding, Chunyan, "Physician-Patient Relationship v. Consumer–Provider Relationship: Lifting the Veil of the Debate" [醫患關係與消費者–經營者關係: 揭開爭議的面紗], *Journal of Law and Medicine* 14, 2007.

Draper, Heather and Tom Sorell, "Patients' Responsibilities in Medical Ethics," *Bioethics* 16(4), 2002.

Eckholm, Erik, "SARS in Beijing: The Unraveling of a Cover-Up," in Arthur Kleinman and James L. Watson, eds., *SARS in China: Prelude to Pandemic?*, Stanford, CA: Stanford University Press, 2005.

Emanuel, Ezekiel and Linda L. Emanuel, "What Is Accountability in Health Care?," *Annals of Internal Medicine* 124(2), 1996.

ESC Committee, General Comment No. 14: The Right to Highest Attainable Standard of Health, E/C.12/2000/4, August 11, 2000, paragraph 43(a)–(f), http://undocs.org/E/C.12/2000/4.

———, General Comment No. 3: The Nature of States Parties' Obligations, E/1991/23, annex III, December 14, 1990, paragraph 10, http://undocs.org/E/1991/23 (SUPP).

Evans, Martyn, "Do Patients Have Duties," *Journal of Medical Ethics* 33(12), 2007.

Fan, Ruiping and Benfu Li, "Truth Telling in Medicine: The Confucian View," *The Journal of Medicine and Philosophy: A Forum for Bioethics and Philosophy of Medicine* 29(2), 2004.

Fan, Ruiping, *Reconstructionist Confucianism: Rethinking Morality After the West*, Dordrecht: Springer Netherlands, 2010.

Fang, Xiaoping, *Barefoot Doctors and Western Medicine in China*, Rochester, NY: University of Rochester Press, 2012.

Farquhar, Judith, "Market Magic: Getting Rich and Getting Personal in Medicine After Mao," *American Ethnologist* 23(2), 1996.

Fidler, David, *SARS, Governance and the Globalization of Disease*, London: Palgrave Macmillan, 2004.

Finnis, John, *Natural Law and Natural Rights*, Oxford; New York: Oxford University Press, 2011.

Fu, Hongqiao, Ling Li, Mingqiang Li, et al. "An Evaluation of Systemic Reforms of Public Hospitals: The Sanming Model in China," *Health Policy and Planning* 32, 2017.

Fu, Hualing, "Politicized Challenges, Depoliticized Responses: Political Monitoring in China's Transitions," *University of Hong Kong Faculty of Law Research Paper 2013/014*, 2013.

———, "The Varieties of Law," https://lawprofessors.typepad.com/china_law_prof_blog/2011/06/fu-hualing-on-the-varieties-of-law.html.

Fukuyama, Francis, "The Pandemic and Political Order," *Foreign Affairs* 99, 2020, https://www.foreignaffairs.com/articles/world/2020-06-09/pandemic-and-political-order.

———, *State-building: Governance and World Order in the 21st Century*, Ithaca, NY: Cornell University Press, 2019.

———, *The Origins of Political Order: From Prehuman Times to the French Revolution*, New York, NY: Farrar, Straus and Giroux 2012.

Gao, Qiang, "Executive Vice Minister of Health Gao Qiang and Others Answer Questions on the Prevention and Treatment of SARS" [衛生部常務副部長高強等就非典防治情況答問], http://news.enorth.com.cn/system/2003/04/21/000547490.shtml.

Global Times, "Doctors Induce Patients to Place Heart Stents" [醫生誘導患者放置心臟支架: 國外用3個國內用10個], https://china.huanqiu.com/article/9CaKrnK1Flk.

Goodrich, Peter, *Reading the Law: A Critical Introduction to Legal Method and Critiques*, New York, NY: Blackwell, 1986.

Gostin, Lawrence, "Public Health Law: A Renaissance," *The Journal Law, Medicine & Ethics* 30(2), 2002.

———, "The Human Right to Health: A Right to the 'Highest Attainable Standard of Health'," *The Hastings Center Report* 31(2), 2001.

Gostin, Lawrence and Lindsay F. Wiley, *Public Health Law: Power, Duty, Restraint*, Berkeley: University of California Press, 2016.

Gross, Miriam, *Farewell to the God of Plague: Chairman Mao's Campaign to Deworm China*, Oakland, CA: University of California Press, 2016.

Gu, Edward and Imogen Page-Jarrett, "The Top-Level Design of Social Health Insurance Reforms in China: Towards Universal Coverage, Improved Benefit Design, and Smart Payment Methods," *Journal of Chinese Governance* 3(3), 2018.

Gu, Edward and Lantian Li, "Crippled Community Governance and Suppressed Scientific/Professional Communities: A Critical Assessment of Failed Early Warning for the Covid-19 Outbreak in China," *Journal of Chinese Governance* 5(2), 2020.

Gu, Xin, "New National Health Care Reform Enters Critical Stage" [全國新醫改進入關鍵階段], *Social Blue Book*, 2011.

Harrington, John, *Towards a Rhetoric of Medical Law: Against Ethics*, Abingdon, Oxon: Routledge, 2016.

He, Alex Jingwei and Jiwei Qian, "Hospitals' Responses to Administrative Cost-Containment Policy in Urban China: The Case of Fujian Province," *China Quarterly* 216, 2013.

———, "Explaining Medical Disputes in Chinese Public Hospitals: The Doctor-Patient Relationship and Its Implications for Health Policy Reforms," *Health, Economy, Policy and Law* 11, 2016.

He, Alex Jingwei, "Combating Healthcare Cost Inflation with Concerted Administrative Actions in a Chinese Province," *Public Administration and Development* 31, 2011.

———, "Manoeuvring Within a Fragmented Bureaucracy: Policy Entrepreneurship in China's Local Healthcare Reform," *China Quarterly* 236, 2018.

———, "China's Ongoing Public Hospital Reform: Initiatives, Constraints and Prospect," *Journal of Asian Public Policy* 4(3), 2011.

———, "Combating Healthcare Cost Inflation with Concerted Administrative Actions in a Chinese Province," *Public Administration and Development* 31(3), 2011.

He, Alex Jingwei, Yuda Shi and Hongdou Liu, "Crisis Governance, Chinese Style: Distinctive Features of China's Response to the Covid-19 Pandemic," *Policy Design and Practice* 3(3), 2020.

He, Zhaoxiong, Chen Lixing, eds., *Introduction to Medical Ethics* [醫學倫理學概論], Nanjing: Jiangsu Science and Technology Publishing House, 1985.

Henaghan, Mark, *Health Professionals and Trust: The Cure for Healthcare Law and Policy*, London: Routledge-Cvendish, 2011.

Hesketh, Therese and Wei Xing Zhu, "Health in China: The Healthcare Market," *BMJ* 314(7094), 1997.

Heymann, David L. and Guenael Rodier, "SARS: Lessons from a New Disease," *Learning from SARS: Preparing for the Next Disease Outbreak*, Washington, DC: National Academies Press, 2004.

Hisao, William, "The Chinese Health Care System: Lessons for Other Nations," *Social Science & Medicine* 41, 1995.

Holton, Richard, "Deciding to Trust, Coming to Believe," *Australasian Journal of Philosophy* 72, 1994.

Huang, Yanzhong, *Governing Health in Contemporary China*, Milton Park, Abingdon, Oxon; New York: Routledge, 2013.

Jian Kangbao, December 12, 1993, Beijing.

Kaufman, Joan, "SARS and China's Health-Care Response: Better to be Both Red and Expert!," in Arthur Kleinman and James L. Watson, eds., *SARS in China: Prelude to Pandemic?*, Stanford, CA: Stanford University Press, 2005.

Khalil, Lydia, "Digital Authoritarianism, China and Covid," *Lowy Institute Analysis*, https://www.lowyinstitute.org/publications/digital-authoritarianism-china-and-covid; https://www.nortonrosefulbright.com/en-cn/knowledge/publications/d7a9a296/contact-tracing-apps-a-new-world-for-data-privacy.

King, Jeff, *Judging Social Rights*, Cambridge: Cambridge University Press, 2012.

Kleinman, Arthur, "Caregiving as Moral Experience," *The Lancet* 380(9853), 2012.

———, "Caregiving: Its Role in Medicine and Society in America and China," *Ageing International* 35, 2010.

———, "Catastrophe and Caregiving: The Failure of Medicine as an Art," *The Lancet* 371(9606), 2008.

Kleinman, Arthur, Veena Das and Margaret Lock, eds., *Social Suffering*, Berkeley: University of California Press, 1997.

Li, Heng, Xiangcheng Wu, Tao Sun, et al., "Claims, Liabilities, Injures and Compensation Payments of Medical Malpractice Litigation Cases in China from 1998 to 2011," *BMC Health Services Research* 14, 2014.

Li, Keqiang, "Continue to Deepen the Healthcare Reform, Promote the Establishment of the Medical and Health System that Suits the National Conditions and Benefits All the People" [不斷深化醫改 推動建立符合國情惠及全民的醫藥衛生體制], *Seeking Truth* 22, 2011.

Li, Rui, *Personal Experience of Great Leap Forward* [大躍進親歷記], Haikou: Nanfang Chubanshe, 1999.

Lieberthal, Kenneth and Michel Oksenberg, *Policy Making in China: Leaders, Structures, and Processes*, Princeton, NJ: Princeton University Press, 1988.

Liebman, Benjamin, "Malpractice Mobs: Medical Dispute Resolution in China," *Columbia Law Review* 113, 2013.

———, "Law in the Shadow of Violence: Can Law Help to Improve Doctor-Patient Trust in China?," *Columbia Journal of Asian Law* 30, 2016.

———, "Legal Reform: China's Law-Stability Paradox," *Daedalus* 143(2), 2014.

Liming Li, Hua Wang, Xiaofeng Liang, et al., "Yiqing Zaoqi, Jibing Yufangkongzhi Tixi Shisheng Yuanyin Hezai?," [疫情早期, 疾病預防控制體系失聲原因何在?], *Intellectual*, http://zhishifenzi.com/depth/depth/8392.html.

Liu, Xingzhu and William C.L. Hsiao, "The Cost Escalation of Social Health Insurance Plans in China: Its Implication for Public Policy," *Social Science & Medicine* 41(8), 1995.

Liu, Yuanli, "China's Public Health-Care System: Facing the Challenges," *Bulletin of the World Health Organization* 82(7), 2004.

Lucas, AnElissa, "Changing Medical Models in China: Organizational Options or Obstacles?," *The China Quarterly* 83, 1980, pp. 461–9.

Lumann, Niklas, *Trust and Power: Two Works by Niklas Luhmann, Chichester*, New York, Brisbane, Toronto: John Wiley & Sons, 1982.

Mann, Michael, *States, War and Capitalism: Studies in Political Economy*, Oxford: Blackwell, 1988.

Mao, Zedong and Zhou Enlai, "Selected Literature of Mao Zedong and Zhou Enlai on Epidemic Control and Medical Care Work," *Literature of Chinese Communist Party* [黨的文獻] 5, 2003.

Marsh, Stephen and Mark Dibben, "Trust, Untrust, Distrust and Mistrust—An Exploration of the Dark(er) Side," in P. Hermann, V. Issarny, S. Shui, eds., *Trust Management*, Berlin: Springer, 2005.

Marshall, Thomas Humphrey, "Citizenship and Social Class," in Thomas Humphrey Marshall and T. Bottomore, eds., *Citizenship and Social Class*, London: Pluto Press, 1992.

Measures of Fujian Province to Implement "the Law of the People's Republic of China on the Consumer Rights and Interests Protection" [福建省實施《中華人民共和國消費者權益保護法》辦法].

Measures of Zhejiang Province to Implement "the Law of the People's Republic of China on the Consumer Rights and Interests Protection" [浙江省實施《中華人民共和國消費者權益保護法》辦法].

Ministry of Health, "Regulation on Medical Work" [醫院工作制度].

Ministry of Health, "Rules for Implementing the Regulation on Medical Institutions" [醫療機構管理條例實施細則].

Miriam, Gross, *Farewell to the God of Plague: Chairman Mao's Campaign to Deworm China*, Oakland, CA: University of California Press, 2016.

Munger, Frank, "Inquiry and Activism in Law and Society," *Law and Society Review* 35(1), 2001.

National Health Commission, "Notice on the Issuance of the Recent Work Program for the Prevention and Control of Pneumonia with Novel Coronavirus Infection" [關於印發近期防控新型冠狀病毒感染的肺炎工

作方案的通知], http://www.nhc.gov.cn/xcs/zhengcwj/202001/808bbf75e5ce415aa19f74c78ddc653f.shtml.

New Hunan, "New Crown Vaccination Program Determined! Health Commission: National Vaccination in a Two-Step Program" [新冠疫苗接種方案確定! 衛健委: 全國接種疫苗分兩步方案], https://hunan.voc.com.cn/xhn/article/202012/202012191037322076.html.

Newdick, Christopher, "Promoting Access and Equity in Health: Assessing the National Health Service in England," in Colleen M. Flood and Aeyal M. Gross, eds., *The Right to Health at the Public/Private Divide: A Global Comparative Study*, New York: Cambridge University Press, 2014.

Newdick, Christopher, *Who Should We Treat? Rights, Rationing and Resources*, Oxford: Oxford University Press, 2005.

Nguyen, Trang (Mae), "Vietnam's Astonishing Success at Curbing Covid-19 Outbreaks," *The Regulatory Review—Opinion*, 2020.

Nie, Jing-Bao, "Is Informed Consent Not Applicable to China? Intellectual Flaws of the 'Cultural Difference Argument'," *Formosan Journal of Medical Humanities* 2(2), 2001.

———, *Medical Ethics in China: A Transcultural Interpretation*, London: Routledge, 2013.

Nie, Jing-Bao, Lun Li, Grant Gillett, Joseph D. Tucker and Arthur Kleinman, "The Crisis of Patient-Physician Trust and Bioethics: Lessons and Inspirations from China," *Developing World Bioethics* 18(1), 2018.

Nie, Jing-Bao, Yu Cheng, Xiang Zou, et al., "The Vicious Circle of Patient-Physician Mistrust in China: Health Professionals' Perspectives, Institutional Conflict of Interest, and Building Trust Through Medical Professionalism," *Developing World Bioethics* 18(1), 2018.

Ning, Yan, Ran Ren and Gerad Nkengurutse, "China's Model to Combat the Covid-19 Epidemic: A Public Health Emergency Governance Approach," *Global Health Research and Policy* 5(1), 2020.

Noddings, Nel, *Educating Moral People: A Caring Alternative to Character Education*, New York: Teachers College Press, 2002.

Notice by the Enforcement Bureau of the Supreme People's Court of Matters Concerning Effectively Conducting the Enforcement Work During the Period of Prevention and Control of the Outbreak of Novel Coronavirus Pneumonia [最高人民法院執行局關於做好防控新型冠狀病毒肺炎疫情期間執行工作相關事項的通知].

Notice by the Supreme People's Court of Strengthening and Regulating the Online Litigation Work During the Period of Prevention and Control of the Covid-19 Outbreak [最高人民法院關於新冠肺炎疫情防控期間加強和規範線上訴訟工作的通知].

Notice of the State Council on Issuing the Plan on Recent Priorities in Carrying Out the Reform of Health Care System (2009–2011) [國務院關於印發醫藥衛生體制改革近期重點實施方案 (2009–2011年) 的通知].

O'Neill, Onora, "Women's Rights: Whose Obligations?," in *Bounds of Justice*, Cambridge; New York: Cambridge University Press, 2000.

———, *Bounds of Justice*, Cambridge; New York: Cambridge University Press, 2000.

———, "The Dark Side of Human Rights," *International Affairs* 81(2), 2005.

Opinions of the Central Committee of the Communist Party of China and the State Council on Deepening the Reform of the Medical and Health System [中共中央國務院關於深化醫藥衛生體制改革的意見].

Pan, Xiao, "Realising the Right to Health: A Comparative Study of South Africa, the United States and China'," H*ong Kong Law Journal* 45, 2015.

Pang, Mei-Che Samantha, "Protective Truthfulness: The Chinese Way of Safeguarding Patients in informed Treatment Decisions," *Journal of Medical Ethics* 25.

Peerenboom, Randall, "A Tale of Two Judiciaries: Judicial Enforcement of Economic and Social Rights in China and India," in Surya Deva, ed., *Socio-Economic Rights in Emerging Free Markets Comparative Insights from India and China*, Abingdon, Oxon: Routledge, 2016.

Peng, Fujun, Lei Tu, Yongshi Yang, et al., "Management and Treatment of COVID-19: The Chinese Experience," *Canadian Journal of Cardiology* 36(6), 2020.

Peng, Jia and Shujuan Yang, "China Needs a National Intelligent Syndromic Surveillance System," *Nature Medicine* 26(7), 2020.

People's Daily Online, "National Health Insurance Bureau: People-Centered, Effective Protection of Patients' Medical Costs" [國家醫保局: 以人民為中心, 切實保障患者醫療費用], http://society.people.com.cn/n1/2020/0329/c1008-31652667.html.

———, "Why Should We Adhere to the Comprehensive Rule of Law?" [為什麼要堅持全面依法治國], http://cpc.people.com.cn/n1/2017/1130/c415067-29677669.html.

Perkins, Dwight and Shahid Yusuf, *Rural Development in China*, Baltimore: Johns Hopkins University Press, 1984.

Pilly, Anashri, "Judicial Activism and the Indian Supreme Court: Lessons for Economic and Social Rights Adjudication," in Liora Lazarus, Christopher McCrudden and Nigel Bowles, *Reasoning Rights: Comparative Judicial Engagement*, Oxford: Hart Publishing, 2014.

Pomfret, John, "China's Slow Reaction to Fast-Moving Illness, *Washington Post*, April 3, 2003, https://www.washingtonpost.com/archive/politics/2003/04/03/chinas-slow-reaction-to-fast-moving-illness/4eac88ab-3b92-4399-8d62-545efc975bc4/.

Qiu, Renzong and Feng Jianmei, *Patients' Rights* [病人的權利], Beijing: Medical University and Peking Union Medical College, 1996.

Qiu, Renzong, "Philosophy of Medicine in China (1939–1980)," *Theoretical Medicine and Bioethics* 3(1), 1982.

Ramcharan, Bertrand, "Implementation of the International Covenant on Economic, Social and Cultural Rights," *Netherlands International Law Review* 23(2), 1976.

Ramesh, Mit, Xun Wu and Alex Jingwei He, "Health Governance and Healthcare Reforms in China," *Health Policy and Planning* 29(6), 2014.

Raposo, Vera Lúcia, "Lost in 'Culturation': Medical Informed Consent in China (from a Western Perspective)," *Medicine, Health Care and Philosophy* 22, 2019.

Raz, Joseph, "On the Nature of Rights," *Mind* 93(370), 1984.

Reiser, Stanley Joel, *Technological Medicine: The Changing World of Doctors and Patients*, New York: Cambridge University Press, 2009.

Ruger, Jennifer, "Toward a Theory of a Right to Health: Capability and Incompletely Theorized Agreements," *Yale Journal of Law & the Humanities* 18(2), 2006.

Ruth, Rogaski, "Nature, Annihilation, and Modernity: China's Korean War Germ-Warfare Experience," *Journal of Asian Studies* 61(2), 2002.

Sathe, Satyaranjan Purushottam, *Judicial Activism in India*, New Delhi: Oxford University Press, 2003.

Scheid, Volker, *Chinese Medicine in Contemporary China: Plurality and Synthesis*, Durham, NC: Duke University Press, 2002.

Schurmann, Franz, *Ideology and Organization in Communist China*, Berkeley, CA: University of California Press, 1968.

Schwartz, Jonathan, R. Gregory Evans and Sarah Greenberg, "Evolution of Health Provision in PreSars China," *China Review*, 2007.

Scott, James, *Seeing Like a State: How Certain Schemes to Improve the Human Condition Have Failed*, New Haven, CT: Yale University Press, 1998.

Shu, Meijun and Jiarui Li, "Health Digital Technology in COVID-19 Pandemic: Experience from China," *BMJ Innovations* 6(4), 2020.

Sohu News, "Central leadership group for the first time disclosed! 11 ministerial-level cadres in Hubei front-line coordination and command," [中央領導組首次披露!11位部級幹部在湖北一線協調指揮], https://www.sohu.com/a/378422340_120053683.

Sohu News, Wuhan to promote the policy "all patients should be collected", how to do? What is the difficulty? [武漢推進"應收盡收", 如何做?難在哪?], https://www.sohu.com/a/371492993_118392.

Southern Weekly, "Wuhan 'collection as much as possible' where is the difficulty" ["武漢'應收盡收'難在何處"], http://www.infzm.com/contents/177054.

Standing Committee of the National People's Congress, Law on Practicing Doctors of the People's Republic of China [中華人民共和國執業醫師法].
Stern, Jessica, "Dreaded Risks and the Control of Biological Weapons," *International Security* 27(3), Winter 2002/2003.
Sun, Shuangyi, Zhen Xie, Keting Yu, Bingqian Jiang, Siwei Zheng and Xiaoting Pan, "COVID-19 and Healthcare System in China: Challenges and Progression for a Sustainable Future," *Globalization and Health* 17, 2021.
Swedberg, Richard ed., *Joseph A. Schumpeter: The Economics and Sociology of Capitalism*, Princeton University Press, 2020.
Tan, Kevin Y. L. "Singapore's Regulatory Response to Covid-19," *Regulation Review—Opinion*, 2020.
Tao, Julia, "Confucian Trust, Market and Health Care Reform," in J. Tao Lai Po-wah, eds., *China: Bioethics, Trust, and the Challenge of the Market*, Springer Science & Business Media, 2008.
Tasioulas, John and Effy Vayena, "Just Global Health: Integrating Human Rights and Common Goods," in Thom Brooks, *The Oxford Handbook of Global Justice*, Oxford: Oxford University Press, 2020.
Tauber, Alfred, "In Search of Medicine's Moral Glue," *American Journal of Bioethics* 6(1), 2006.
Tobin, John, *The Right to Health in International Law*, Oxford; New York: Oxford University Press, 2012.
Tsou, Tang, "Interpreting the Revolution in China: Macrohistory and Micromechanisms," *Modern China* 26(2), 2000.
Tucker, Joseph D., Bonnie Wong, Jing-Bao Nie and Arthur Kleinman, "Rebuilding Patient–Physician Trust in China," *The Lancet* 388, 2016.
Veitch, Kenneth, "Obligation and the Changing Nature of Publicly Funded Healthcare," *Medical Law Review* 27(2), 2019.
Veitch, Scott, "Common Good No More? Some Jurisprudential Reflections on European (Dis)Integration," in Johan van der Walt and Jeffrey Ellsworth, *Constitutional Sovereignty and Social Solidarity in Europe*, Germany: Nomos, 2015.
———, "The Sense of Obligation," *Jurisprudence* 8(3), 2017.
———, *Law and Irresponsibility: On the Legitimation of Human Suffering*, Abingdon; New York: Routledge-Cavendish, 2007.
———, *Obligations: New Trajectories in Law*, Abingdon, Oxon; New York, NY: Routledge, 2021.
Vinen, Richard, *Thatcher's Britain: The Politics and Social Upheaval of the 1980s*, London: Simon & Schuster, Limited, 2010.
Waldron, Jeremy, "Duty-Bearers for Positive Rights," *NYU School of Law, Public Law Research Paper No. 14–58*, 2014.
———, "Rights in Conflict," *Ethics* 99(3), 1989.
———, "The Concept and the Rule of Law," *Georgia Law Review* 43(1), 2008.

Wang, Shaoguang and Peng Fan, *The Chinese Model of Consensus Decision-Making: A Case Study of Healthcare Reform* [中國式共識型決策: "開門"與"磨合"], Beijing: China People's University Press, 2013.

Wang, Shaoguang, "Adapting by Learning: The Evolution of China's Rural Health Care Financing," *Modern China* 35, 2009.

———, "China's Double Movement in Health Care," *Socialist Register* 46, 2010.

———, "China's Health System: From Crisis to Opportunity," *Yale-China Health Journal* 3, 2004.

Wang, Zhu and Ken Oliphant, "Yangge Dance: The Rhythm of Liability for Medical Malpractice in the People's Republic of China," *Chicago-Kent Law Review* 87(1), 2012.

Wei, Furong, Meng Du and Yifan Zhang, "Wuhan Yiqing Chuqi, Wangluo Zhibao Xitong Weihe Shiling" [武漢疫情初期, 網路直報系統為何失靈], Phoenix New Media, https://news.ifeng.com/c/7uqH6A5PWt7.

Wei, Yingmin, *New Ethics Teaching* [新倫理學教程], Beijing: Beijing University Press, 2000.

Wei, Yujun, Zhonghua Ye, Meng Cui and Xiaokun Wei, "Covid-19 Prevention and Control in China: Grid Governance," *Journal of Public Health* 43(1), 2021.

White, Sydney D., "From 'Barefoot Doctor' to 'Village Doctor' in Tiger Springs Village: A Case Study of Rural Health Care Transformations in Socialist China," *Human Organization* 57(4), 1998.

World Health Organization and the United Nations Children's Fund, "Primary Health Care: A Joint Report by the Director-General of the World Health Organization and the Executive Director of the United Nations Children's Fund," International Conference on Primary Health Care, Alma-Ata, USSR, September 1978.

World Health Organization, "Preamble to the Constitution of the World Health Organization".

Worsley, Peter, "Non-Western Medical Systems," *Annual Review of Anthropology* 11(1), 1982.

Wu, Jun, Jian Wang, Stephen Nicholas, et al. "Application of Big Data Technology for COVID-19 Prevention and Control in China: Lessons and Recommendations," *Journal of Medical Internet Research* 22(10), 2020.

Xi, Chao and Lixin Yang, "Medical Liability Laws in China: The Tale of Two Regimes, *Tort Law Review* 19(2), 2011.

Xinhua News, "China Focus: China Inaugurates National Administration of Disease Prevention and Control," http://www.xinhuanet.com/english/2021-05/13/c_139943875.htm.

———, "Xi Focus: Chronicle of Xi's Leadership in China's War Against Coronavirus," http://www.xinhuanet.com/english/2020-09/07/c_139349538.htm.

Xu, Yunbei, "Carrying Out the Great People's Health Work" [開展偉大的人民衛生工作], *Hongqi* 6, 1960.

Yan Longming and Others v Zhuhai Hospital of Guangdong Provincial Hospital of Traditional Chinese Medicine [嚴龍明等與廣東省中醫院珠海醫院非醫療事故損害賠償糾紛上訴案].

Yan, Yunxiang, "The Changing Moral Landscape," in Arthur Kleinman, Yunxiang Yan, Jing Jun, et al., eds., *Deep China: The Moral Life of the Person*, Berkeley: University of California Press, 2011.

———, "The Ethics and Politics of Patient-Physician Mistrust in Contemporary China," *Developing World Bioethics* 18, 2018.

Yang, Lixin and Yuan Xueshi, "On the Medical Organization's Tort Liability of Violating the Obligation of Informed Consent" [論醫療機構違反告知義務的醫療侵權責任], *Hebei Law Science* 12 [河北法學], 2006.

Yang, Nianqun, *Remaking the 'Patient': The Politics of Space in the Conflict Between Chinese and Western Medicine 1832–1985* [再造"病人": 中西醫衝突下的空間政治], Beijing: Beijing Renmin University Press.

Yip, Ka-che, *Health and National Reconstruction in Nationalist China, the Development of Modern Health Services, 1928–1937*, Ann Arbor, MI: Association for Asian Studies, 1995.

Yip, Winnie and William C. Hsiao, "The Chinese Health System at a Crossroads," *Health Affairs* 27(2), 2008.

Yu, Zeyuan, "Shenzhen Becomes the First Region in China to Implement End-of-Life Medical Care Legislation" [深圳成中國首個實現生前預囑立法地區], https://www.zaobao.com.sg/news/china/story20220705-1289640.

Zhan, Jifu, *Comprehensive Reform of Public Hospitals in Sanming City* [三明市公立醫院綜合改革], Fuzhou: Fujian People's Press, 2014.

Zhang, Hongzhu, Zhaoxiong He and Lianzhuang Chi, *A Survey of Chinese Foreign Medical Moral Standards* [中外醫德規範通覽], Tianjin: Tianjin Ancient Books Press, 2000.

Zhang, Kaining, Yiqun Wen and Ping Liang, *From Barefoot Doctors to Village Doctors* [從赤腳醫生到鄉村醫生], Kunming: Yunnan People's Press.

Zhang, Taisu, "China's Turn Toward Law," *Virginia Journal of International Law* 59, 2019.

Zhao, Xiju, "Chinese Medical Negligence Law: How to Distinguish and Accommodate Common Law Principles?," in Lei Chen and C.H. (Remco) van Rhee, eds., *Towards a Chinese Civil Code: Comparative and Historical Perspectives*, Leiden: Brill Nijhoff Publisher, 2012.

Zhao, Xiju, *Study on Medical Law* [醫事法研究], Beijing: Law Press China, 2008.

———, *The Duty of Medical Practitioners and CAM/TCM Practitioners to Inform Competent Adult Patients About Alternatives*, Heidelberg, Germany: Springer, 2013.

Zhong, Raymond, Paul Mozur and Aaron Krolik, "Leaked Documents Show How China's Army of Paid Internet Trolls Helped Censor the Coronavirus," *ProPublica & New York Times*, https://www.propublica.org/article/leaked-documents-show-how-chinas-army-of-paid-internet-trolls-helped-censor-the-coronavirus.

Zhu, Wang and Ken Oliphant, "Yangge Dance: The Rhythm of Liability for Medical Malpractice in the People's Republic of China," *Chicago-Kent Law Review* 87(1), 2012.

Zhu, Wei, *Informed Consent in Bioethics* [生命倫理中的知情同意], Shanghai: Fudan University Press, 2009.

Zou, Xiang, Yu Cheng and Jing-Bao Nie, "The Social Practice of Medical Guanxi (Personal Connections) and Patient-Physician Trust in China: An Anthropological and Ethical Study," *Developing World Bioethics* 18(1), 2018.

Index

L. Jia, *Obligation*, IPP Studies in the Frontiers of China's Public Policy,
https://doi.org/10.1007/978-981-99-6437-6

SPRINGER NATURE

GPSR Compliance

The European Union's (EU) General Product Safety Regulation (GPSR) is a set of rules that requires consumer products to be safe and our obligations to ensure this.

If you have any concerns about our products, you can contact us on ProductSafety@springernature.com

In case Publisher is established outside the EU, the EU authorized representative is:

Springer Nature Customer Service Center GmbH
Europaplatz 3
69115 Heidelberg, Germany